Studies in Alternative Therapy 4

Lifestyle and Medical Paradigms

Studies in Alternative Therapy 4

Lifestyle

and

Medical Paradigms

Edited by

Søren Gosvig Olesen, Bent Eikard

Palle Gad & Erling Høg

INRAT

Odense University Press

Studies in Alternative Therapy 4 is published in
cooperation with the International Network for
Research on Alternative Therapies (INRAT) and
sponsored by the Danish Research Council
for the Humanities (SHF).

© The Authors and Odense University Press 1997
Printed by Narayana Press, Gylling, Denmark
Cover by Ulla Poulsen Precht
ISBN 87-7838-207-6

Contents

Introduction

Søren Gosvig Olesen et al.	Introduction: Lifestyle and Medical Paradigms	7

Lifestyle   9

Jørgen Ø. Andersen	Lifestyles, Consumption and Alternative Therapies	11
Dirk Richter	Lifestyles – Different Cultural Pathways to Alternative Treatment	27
Adrian Furnham	Lifestyle, Beliefs and Value Systems, and Complementary Medicine	43
Nelly Tsouyopoulos	Coping with Emotions and Stress of Life	71
David Aldridge	Lifestyle, Charismatic Ideology and a Praxis Aesthetic	81

Medical Paradigms   101

Palle Gad	Quality in Clinical Holistic Medicine – Criteria, Assessment and Handling	103
Søren Brier	The Self-organization of Knowledge: Paradigms of Knowledge and their Role in the Decision of what Counts as Legitimate Medical Practice	112
Laila Launsø	The Connection between the Scope of Diagnosis and the User's Scope of Action – Empirical Findings and Theoretical Perspectives	136
Ane Bodil Søgaard	Organic Agriculture and Alternative Medicine: Parallels and Paradigms	150

Methodology 165

Mary Ryan-Thorup	Methodologies along a Spectrum: From the Randomized Controlled Trial to Post-Modern Queries	167
Jørgen Ø. Andersen et al.	Abstracts on Methodology	181
Helle Johannessen et al.	INRAT – a network project for research on alternative therapies	205

List of contributors 220

Introduction:
Lifestyle and Medical Paradigms

by Søren Gosvig Olesen, Bent Eikard, Palle Gad & Erling Høg

The present volume of *Studies in Alternative Therapy* originated at the fourth and final international INRAT seminar.[1] Unlike previous seminars, there were no formal presentation of papers, but the seminar was organized as discussion groups, since the participants were prepared, having received the seminar papers weeks in advance. The volume here contains the final versions of these papers. A draft version of the chapter on methodology included here was also discussed at the seminar. Participants' contributions to the discussion in the form of methodology abstracts have been integrated and cited in the final version.

The book presents two major themes, *lifestyle* and *medical paradigms*. Both themes are shaped by an interdisciplinary approach. Taking *lifestyle* as a point of departure for describing the use and users of alternative therapies takes research beyond the traditional economic and social categories of explanation. By designating the *style* as a decisive factor we suggest that alternative treatment can be viewed as a cultural phenomenon by which people may or may not find self-identification. Alternative treatment is predominantly perceived as creating identity, indicating by that the personal identity is crucial, including whatever may be imaginary. The concept of lifestyle is hardly a ponderous, or well-established, scientific category, and it may therefore be well suited for apprehending the phenomenon of alternative treatment in all its hovering complexity.

Under the heading of *Medical Paradigms* we try to characterize the differences between established and alternative treatment. Starting from the conven-

---

[1] The seminar "Lifestyle, Medical Paradigms and Methodology in Research on Alternative Therapies" took place in Værløse, Denmark, during the days November 1-3, 1996. Forty-three researchers representing institutions of higher education in Austria, California, Denmark, England, Germany, Norway, Sweden and Switzerland participated in the seminar. Friday, November 1, was preset for a presentation and discussion of papers distributed before the seminar, Saturday, November 2, for a methodological discussion and for workshops on the issue of "After INRAT," while Sunday, November 3, was assigned to the INRAT organizing committee for evaluating the results of the network project and considering future research activities.

tional idea of a scientific paradigm, the established medical treatment can be linked to the mathematically founded natural science. This foundation is often generalized as a scientific ideal, but it should be clear that such an ideal creates distortion when applied to alternative treatment. However, it is less clear which paradigm to apply in characterizing alternative treatment. Experimentally, we could start with the techniques of holography, or the philosophical directions that have been dominating in epistemological discussions, such as phenomenology or hermeneutics. The question of an alternative to established science and treatment could ultimately be a question of the difference between the dominating Western tradition versus Eastern traditions. What possibilities do we have for characterizing a break with traditions?

In the final section of this volume you will find several documents concerning the evaluation and conclusion of the 1993-97 research project INRAT. The initial article in this section discusses problems of methodologies within the research area of alternative therapies. This article is linked to several abstracts on methodology submitted by seminar participants invited to write a few words about their experiences regarding methodology in conducting alternative therapy research. Lastly, we bring you the final report on project INRAT, which the organizing committee submitted to the Research Council of the Humanities, Copenhagen, Denmark. This text is a concluding document in relation to the granting authorities, which offers the reader an insight into the progress of activities within the research network.

As indicated, the publication of *Studies in Alternative Therapy 4* marks the 'end' of the INRAT research network itself. The weary term 'end' should, however, in this context be understood more as a crossroad: The editors and the INRAT working group as a whole hope that the researchers who met at INRAT seminars will continue this in new, yet ongoing, international research connections.

Lifestyle

Lifestyles, Consumption and Alternative Therapies

by Jørgen Østergård Andersen

This paper addresses the point that lifestyle is of intimate import with how a person chooses to define him- or herself, and that a lifestyle is found in the actual practice of individuals. Choosing a lifestyle implies a certain aesthetic style and performance, which is a juggling of internal as well as external dimensions of the personality. Thus choices and decisions on what to choose – and not to choose – in the health-seeking process are twofold. The consumption of alternative therapies reflects on the one hand an *internal* process, i.e., the health-seeking process is motivated by an internal need to be cured; on the other hand, such preferences and decisions are *external* signals which the social network must interpret and react to. Relatives, friends and colleagues may – or may not – legitimize the decision to choose a certain therapy or medical treatment as being the appropriate manner, ethics, personality, identity, social status or lifestyle of the person.

This point came to me while I was performing ethnographic fieldwork among traditional Ayurvedic practitioners and their patients in Sri Lanka. I came to realize that there is no significant difference between the practice of patients, healers and medical doctors in Sri Lanka and in Western Europe and in the USA on a theoretical level of abstraction, where we talk about the construction of identities, the formation of lifestyles, the consumption of medical treatments and therapies and the practice of image-management of healers and doctors. In both places the situation is complex, and though the complexity of knowledge and practice of indigenous medicine in Sri Lanka is very different from the complex situation we find in our postmodern cultures, the need to juggle internal and external processes of the personality is the same. At this fundamental level of human practice and personal needs, we find differences which are too small and subtle to become cultural distinctions.

When we talk about consumption of medical treatment and therapies in Sri Lanka, in the USA, in Denmark, in Germany and in other places, we talk about three kinds of differences. First, we have a cultural difference which is too small and too subtle to be noticed by the recipient. Secondly, we have an appreciable difference which is big enough to be noticed, and therefore evokes a cultural distinction. A third kind of difference is too great and may have a disorganizing effect on the recipient system. In such cases the recipient closes itself to that information which would implement such a difference.

It is the art and craft of social anthropologists like Mary Douglas to talk about the third kind of difference which the social system cannot integrate, since such information disturbs the integrity of the recipient system. Mary Douglas celebrates a perspective which is truly international and modern, since it transcends the local constraints (cf. Mary Douglas 1996: chap. 2: "The Choice Between Gross and Spiritual: Some Medical Preferences").

In this article I would rather focus on a subtle difference which is too small to be appreciated as a cultural distinction. I will talk about the consumption of medical treatment and therapy, and I will focus on the fact that most Danes decide *not* to choose a treatment and choose to *do nothing* about serious symptoms like fatigue, anxiety, pain, depression etc. This practice of *non-doing* is a subtle and unrecognized cultural practice which becomes distinctly different in an anthropological comparison with the cultural practice of the Sinhalese in Sri Lanka.

Lifestyles and Consumption

In postmodern cultures we do not find the kind of struggle between social classes found earlier, and the social identity is no longer primarily formed by class-consciousness. Instead we have the tyranny of cultural differences, and we find a social identity generated by a lifestyle which is not the essence of a social class. These observations do not imply that we are facing the end of poverty and of struggles between social classes and between economic interests; merely that since the 1980s we have been observing a new tendency which is emerging in Western Europe and in the USA, which Gerhard Schulze describes as *Die Erlebnisgeschellschaft* (The Experience Society) (Schulze 1992).

Lifestyle is to be distinguished from social class and social status, though it may stem from both. A given lifestyle may be characteristic of a specific class, status group, or subculture; but since lifestyle is defined in terms of shared preferences and by the set of choices which forms a collective pattern in the society, it is possible, and indeed is often the case, that a lifestyle may be defined over a collectivity that otherwise lacks social and cultural identity. Individuals being conditioned by the same social and economic determinants may have very different lifestyles due to different preferences and different ways of dealing with the social determinants. A lifestyle is found in the actual practice of individuals.

A lifestyle is the *pattern* in which an individual lives and spends his or her time, and it is the *paradigm* which frames a world view of a collectivity which consists of individuals who spend their time in search of meaning or experience which is shared by other individuals.

The collectivity of a lifestyle is formed by shared aesthetic preferences and by choices, since a lifestyle provides a set of cultural distinctions which frames the identity of the individual. Since many individuals share the same *taste*, which organizes the preferences and choices among distinct cultural differences, a collectivity is formed. When an individual chooses to define him or herself within a certain lifestyle, he or she identifies him/herself with a certain taste which is shared by other individuals.

The space of a lifestyle is formed by these shared aesthetic preferences, and a line is drawn between those who belong to a lifestyle and those who do not, since the aesthetic taste – and the decisions about what to choose or not to choose – delineates who belongs to a lifestyle and who does not.

In postmodern cultures the individual is a consumer, who constantly makes decisions about what to choose – and not to choose. By choosing the kind of cultural distinctions which are provided by a lifestyle, the consumer relates him- or herself to an outer world of social life. Consumption is an extension of the individual person into social space, and by the consumption of artifacts, clothes, food etc. the body is extended into social life.

How do these concepts of lifestyle and consumption relate to alternative therapies? I suggest that the consumption of alternative therapies in postmodern cultures should be seen as an extension of the body into social space, like fashion, artifacts, food etc., and that the consumption of therapies should be appreciated as a marking of a lifestyle which establishes a set of cultural distinctions. What I am suggesting is that the health-seeking processes should also be seen as a marking of cultural preferences and lifestyle distinctions – and not only as the outcome of a personal need, or determined by the health-care system.

It is my argument that there is not a simple relationship between body and culture in postmodern cultures. I doubt that it has ever been so that the body simply mirrors a culture, since I have found in traditional Sinhalese culture in Sri Lanka that the relationship between the internal needs of the body and the external world is much more complicated than the simple model of correspondence between body and culture tells us. We must integrate the fact that cultural distinctions and aesthetic preferences have something to say in the relationship between body and culture.

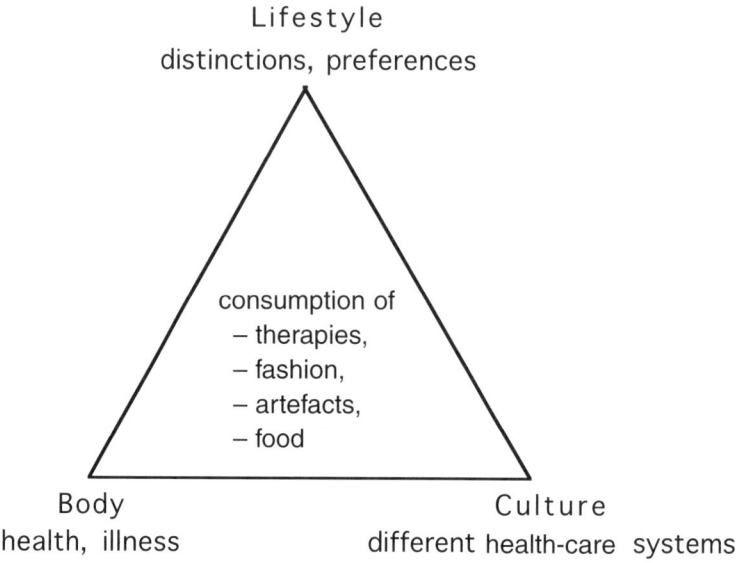

Lifestyles, Networks and Indigenous Medicine in Sri Lanka

What the Ayurvedic practitioners *offer*, and what their patients *use*, is based on an inherently rational set of interactions. Each group assesses its own needs in relation to the availability of services and the social norms of the community. In each case patients and practitioners enter into a dynamic relationship in which the requirements and values of both are negotiated.

Patients do not make decisions on which practitioner to consult based solely on individual illnesses and personal dilemmas. Their lifestyle comes into question, and the kinds of practitioners they go to are social status markers. Questions of social status, of balancing personal concerns with the social identity by which they prefer to be perceived, of pragmatism, of maintaining meaningful frameworks of interaction, and of satisfying medical conventions in the face of the respected traditions in the society influence the decision of patients in Sri Lanka.

Though the Ayurvedic practitioners are devoted to concerns of illness, they are also concerned about questions of social status and of balancing personal concerns with the social identity by which they prefer to be perceived. Their knowledge and medical practice are managed and negotiated, and they are skillful in style-management.

In terms of social criteria – and not medical criteria – higher class and caste divisions are associated with private allopathic care, and the lower ones with indigenous care. Yet medically speaking, most of the population generally consider Ayurvedic medicine to be superior. This distinction between social and medical criteria explains why many people contradict what they actually do when facing an illness, and why many people contradict what they say they do. Various people have various accepted parameters of action.

Medical information is passed through family networks and local-level village networks, and these networks are instrumental in providing primary health care and in circulating current medical knowledge. They gain their knowledge by supplementing information on home remedy with personal experiences with illness. These networks combine several domains of health practice, providing advice, healing and treatments which may be based either on Ayurvedic medicine or allopathy, and in some instances both. These networks mediate social and medical criteria for decisions on curative practice, and they make crucial decisions on behalf of the patient. Medical information is sought from these networks by the patient in the process of seeking health, *before* a decision is taken to consult a professional or folk practitioner.

Ayurveda provides a frame of reference for practitioners, patients and the public in Sri Lanka, and the Sinhalese know a considerable number of herbal remedies and their basic "qualities". The Sinhalese give expression to the humoural theory associated with Ayurveda in their daily conversations. Ayurveda also provides a framework for healthy behaviour and therefore constitutes a set of principles guiding day-to-day conduct: eating, bathing, sleeping, making love etc. So, Ayurveda is not merely a curative system but a preventive one as well, and the Ayurvedic practitioner has no total monopoly over knowledge and action. For instance, the afflicted, under the guidance of their close relatives or friends, may try many home remedies before consulting an Ayurvedic practitioner. Ayurveda is generally thought to be a way of life and a framework for remaining healthy. A Sinhalese person has to consult a folk or professional specialist only when the illness is too complex to be comprehended by laymen, and when the situation requires a specialist for diagnosis and treatment.

This situation has not been subjected to the modernizing forces during the long period of colonial rule in Sri Lanka, and what is important to recognize is that the introduction of Western, allopathic medicine and its propagation during the later part of the British rule and thereafter has not altered the relationship between the traditional Ayurvedic practitioners, their patients, the herbal medicine prescribed and the public.

During my fieldwork in Sri Lanka in 1994, I studied the knowledge and practice of Ayurvedic practitioners and their patients in Yatinuvara district, and I interviewed 46 practitioners.

A generalized representation of the Ayurvedic practitioners in Yatinuvara district will show that the practitioners neither have a general practice like a Western G.P. (only 6 of the respondents had a general practice like a Western trained medical doctor) nor a single specialty like snakebites or burns or fractures (only 7 of the respondents were such a kind of *parampara veda mahattayo*). Most of the respondents had a general knowledge of Ayurvedic principles, but they were also experts on one or two diseases like children's diseases, fractures, *vata-roga*, *pinasa*, rabies, eye-problems or skin-problems. Most of the practitioners had learned Ayurvedic medicine from a close relative (only 13 of the respondents had been to an Ayurvedic college, and only 7 of these 13 respondents had only been trained at an Ayurvedic college or Ayurvedic school – i.e., only 7 respondents did not learn Ayurveda in a tacit teacher-student relationship, but obtained their medical knowledge from a teaching institution). All respondents collected herbal plants themselves and prepared their own medicine (oils, decoctions, powder or pills). They bought Ayurvedic plant materials (for on average 1500 rupees per month) primarily from the Ayurvedic Cooperation in Kandy. Only one respondent did not buy herbal plant materials, and she collected all the materials herself from her garden and from the forest. Six respondents bought a large quantity of Ayurvedic medicine from the Ayurvedic pharmaceutical industries, which they dispensed to their patients.

All respondents knew at least 125 different herbal plants, and they taught their patients to collect the herbal plants necessary for a cure (only 3 respondents did not ask the patient to collect plants). Most practitioners asked the patients to help them to collect herbal plants for their medicine, which the practitioners prepared and dispensed from their clinics, and only a very few practitioners had "professional" collectors, who collected herbal plant materials regularly and were paid to do so by the practitioners.

Most Ayurvedic practitioners in Yatinuvara district complemented their treatment of Ayurvedic medicine with other forms of healing. Forty of the respondents used mantras or yantras, and 21 used astrology in their clinical work. Twenty-one of the respondents had a contact to a *devela*, which implies spiritual guidance or support from a god. Almost all the Ayurvedic practitioners in Yatinuvara district were in the habit of directing their patients to a Buddhist priest, who could complement or support the healing process of a patient by a prayer to Lord Buddha or by a sacrifice at the Bo-tree.

In Sri Lanka we find local networks, therapeutic actions and interactions between healers and patients, which connect certain herbal plants with other plant materials in a medical practice – i.e., in a medicine which circulates in singular relationships between the practitioners, their patients and the public. A plant is significant only in relation to an actual and concrete medicine. The practitioner who produces the medicine has a localized knowledge which situates the plant in a concrete relationship which the practitioner reproduces by a repetition of the tradition. Medical knowledge and medical practice is *not* about the abstract qualities of the plants, and knowledge is *not* distributed in a top-down descending mental process from abstract principles and theories to a level of actual practice. Knowledge is produced and reproduced in the local networks, and it is circulated in the networks.

Alternative Therapies in USA

Meredith McGuire's representation of alternative therapies in America is based on a thorough study of a well-defined catchment area in New Jersey (McGuire 1988). The study demonstrates the presence of Eastern philosophical and Christian metaphysical concepts and a plurality of alternative healing methods. McGuire reduces the plurality of healing practices into four groups: Christian groups, Metaphysical groups, Eastern Meditation and Human Potential groups and Psychic groups, and she describes the features of these groups: the ideals of health and wellness, the notions of illness and healing, causes of illness, the diagnostic approaches, sources of healing power, healing and health practices, therapeutic success, therapeutic failure and death.

Meredith McGuire's study dissolves the common misconception that alternative medicine functions merely as an alternative healing technique to which people resort when all else fails. McGuire's study found that only a tiny minority of adherents initially came to their alternative healing group or healer out of a need to heal a prior condition. Most adherents were initially attracted by the larger system of beliefs of which health-illness related beliefs and practices are only one part.

Meredith McGuire and her research fellows also studied a fifth type of alternative healing methods: the technique practitioners, those using, for example, shiatsu, the chiropractic method, acupuncture and reflexology. This type was based upon applying a technique, typically in a client-adherent relationship rather than in a group setting. Meredith McGuire argues that many studies of "alternative" or "holistic" healing equate these nonmedical practitioners with the entire alternative healing movement. Various technique practitioners, including acupuncturists, homeopaths and naturopaths, appear to be the main professional alternative healing competition to medical doctors; but there were relatively few respondents in McGuire's study who considered technique practitioners their main form of alternative healing. Rather, they generally viewed the practitioner as providing a limited service.

Meredith McGuire's study reveals that the technique practitioners are only one form of alternative healing. They are competing with the biomedical system, but the adherents of alternative healing practices are more concerned about the metaphysical content of a cosmological system.

Meredith McGuire's study challenges the conception of alternative methods of healing in Denmark, since it changes the perspective concerning technique practitioners, who are considered by Danish sociologists to be the most important representatives of the alternative healing movement. McGuire's study is challenging, since we have to consider whether our sociological research on alternative therapies in Denmark is methodologically biased, because the perspective only focuses on alternative therapies which challenge the biomedical system.

One may object that Meredith McGuire's finding of a plurality of cosmological systems in New Jersey which evoke specific health-illness and body related practices, may be a special case and out of tune with the general tendency in Western Europe and in USA, but I see the postmodern situation of a plurality of metaphysical and cosmological systems described by McGuire, *not* to be particularly American. The practice of alternative healing and therapy and the attachment to metaphysical and cosmological systems, where each of them evokes alternative health-illness related beliefs and practices, is a general movement within the modern, Western world – the so-called 'free world'.

The health-care systems in America and in Denmark are no doubt different; the options for a cure, which a patient may choose in seeking health, may be different; and we may discover small and subtle differences between the religious, spiritual and metaphysical situation in USA and Denmark; but both countries share the same history after 1945, and alternative health-illness beliefs and alternative practices concerning the body are important aspects of this globalizing movement within the free, Western world.

USA and Western Europe share the same process of modernization. I tend to see modernity as a reaction, and I personally believe that modernity is conditioned by the defeat of the Nazi metaphysical system in 1945, and that this global conflict and traumatizing experience of Western civilization has been repeating itself for the last 50 years. Others claim that the modern world became anti-metaphysical after the First World War with the rise of modern art, psychoanalysis etc., and some say that Friedrich Nietzsche in the last century was the first to realize that the modern world must be anti-metaphysical, since God is dead, and all values therefore have to be reevaluated.

Whatever is the case, we are living in an anti-metaphysical world. In comparison with the cosmological order of traditional cultures – like Sinhalese Buddhist cosmology in Sri Lanka (cf. J. Østergård Andersen 1992, 1994) – we are confronted with a strong anti-metaphysical tendency in Western civilization, when we live our lives in our present postmodern cultures. Contemporary philosophy of science and conventional allopathic medicine is extremely anti-metaphysical. But alternative therapies, which evoke a plurality of metaphysical systems, are coexisting with this dominating tendency in our contemporary societies.

I suggest that the split between mainstream philosophy and mainstream medicine on one hand and alternative therapies on the other is constituted by the global conflict of the Second World War. Herbert Schulze observes the same split and conflict, since he distinguished between 'Techniches Wissen' and 'Existentielles Wissen',[1] but he interprets our contemporary history somewhat differently. Schulze argues that technical knowledge is situationalized, and can therefore be judged and evaluated against a clearly defined goal. Existential knowledge, however, is universal in scope and frames the goals, which implies that existential knowledge is unstable and does not have clear-cut criteria which can evaluate the quality of that kind of knowledge.

These two different types of knowledge have developed differently according to Gerhard Schulze (Schulze op. cit.: 223-224). Technical knowledge has become more and more universal, since new techniques have been globalized and are widely circulated – although technical knowledge by definition is bound to concrete situations. Existential knowledge on the other hand, which is global in scope, has lost its significance and has become local knowledge which is circulated in local networks such as groups of friends, within the family, with close relatives, with colleagues – and in the context of alternative therapies.

Most of the healing groups Meredith McGuire has studied circulate existential knowledge, and though the adherents of alternative therapies share the technical knowledge of their countrymen, they indulge in metaphysical systems when they are confronted with an illness, or when they meet their internal needs. But, contrary to the cultural practices of Sinhalese Buddhists in Sri Lanka, such health-body related practices, which are motivated by an internal need to be cured or to experience some internal dimensions of the body and which raise metaphysical questions, are marginalized and subdued by the dominating technological tendency of postmodern cultures.

---

1 Schulze 1992, p. 223: *"Technisches Wissen ist die Gesamtheit der Informationen darüber, wie man möglichst effizient genau definierte Zwecke erreicht. Als Teilmengen sind Expertenwissen und technisches Alltagswissen zu unterscheiden. Existentielles Wissen dagegen betrifft das Leben in seiner Gesamtheit. Es ist nicht instrumentell in einen gegebenen Rahmen eingespannt, sondern der Rahmen selbst."*

Alternative Therapies in Denmark and Consumption of Treatments

I have calculated that the Danes have more than 3.9 million contacts with alternative therapists per year (Østergård Andersen 1995: 17). We do not know the exact numbers of alternative therapists in Denmark, and consequently we do not know the pattern and extent of consumption of alternative therapies here. Sociologists tend to define alternative therapists as practitioners who offer treatments which are alternatives to the medical treatments which are offered by the medical establishment (cf. Laila Launsø 1996a, 1996b and Helle Johannessen 1994). We know something about those whom Meredith McGuire calls 'technique practitioners', but we do not know the amount of healing sessions or group meetings which are not simply duplicating or competing with the medical treatments of the medical establishment, and we do not know the amount of therapies and health-related practices which are related to human growth and spiritual development.

We have more detailed information about the consumption of allopathic medical treatments. We know that Danes have almost thirty million contacts with their three thousand general practitioners, and that 80.3% of the population meet their G.P.s at least once a year – on average 7.2 contacts per year.[2] The general practitioners are "gatekeepers" within the Danish health-care system, and they solve 95% of the complaints directed to them. The rest is channelled to 9,087 medical doctors within the system of hospitals and specialized clinics. One-fifth of these five percent is hospitalized (ibid: 39).

Two percent of the Danes who realize that they are ill and have a symptom of a sickness, and who have reported to DIKE that they have a serious symptom within the last fourteen days, consult an alternative therapist (DIKE 1988). Fifteen percent consult a medical doctor (G.P.), and nineteen percent of these Danes, who feel and realize that they are ill, treat themselves on their own. Seventeen percent use previously prescribed medicine by a G.P., and nine percent treat themselves according to previous advice by a G.P. (Institut for Fremtidsforskning 1994: 43).

Only four percent of those who have reported a symptom, consult a relative or a friend. This is a different practice in comparison with the cultural practice of Sinhalese in Sri Lanka, who live in family networks and local level village networks. An even more striking and significant difference – though small and subtle – is that forty percent of those who are confronted with a symptom in Denmark choose to *do nothing*:

---

2   Danes had 29.3 million contacts with their General Practitioners in 1991, and per 31.12. 1992 there were 3233 G.P.s in Denmark (Institut for Fremtidsforskning 1994: 3, 43).

fatigue	61%	do nothing
common cold	59%	– –
anxiety and nervousness	38%	– –
headache	23%	– –
rash and itching	22%	– –
pain in neck or shoulder	42%	– –
pain in back or lumbar region	40%	– –
pain in stomach	39%	– –
indigestion	36%	– –
shortness of breath	41%	– –
palpitation	45%	– –
light sleeping	46%	– –
depression	43%	– –

Source: DIKE 1988 & Institut for Fremtidsforskning 1994: 30.

I find these figures striking, and in an anthropological perspective it is interesting to observe that only one-fifth of those who feel they are sick seek external help, and almost one-half of those who are sick (40%) choose to do nothing – not even help themselves. The response to certain symptoms like 'fatigue' and 'common cold' by *doing nothing* is up to 61%.

Relatively few Danes (22%) *do nothing* towards symptoms like 'rash' and 'itching', but seek medical advice (34%), and 46% treat themselves on their own or by previously prescribed medicine; and the response toward 'headache' is that only 23% *do nothing*, while 39% find their own way of healing, 23% use previously prescribed medicine and 8% consult a general practitioner. The response toward 'anxiety' and 'nervousness' is somewhat different: 38% respond by *doing nothing*, 9% treat themselves, 26% use previously prescribed medicine and 16% consult a G.P.[3]

Danes' responses to symptoms are very complex, and it could be interesting to identify the responses with various lifestyles; but the DIKE study of Danes' responses to various symptoms only shows the complexity of the situation.

From an anthropological perspective it is a very exotic culture which spends 3,100 million Danish kroner on medical science per year – 1,100 by the Danish government (NASTRA 1995: 29) – and which does not even spend one million on research on alternative therapies. Nobody seems to be concerned about the 40% who feel sick, but choose to do nothing about it, and the 80% who decide not to

---

[3] The figures are for the year 1987, and the study classifies the responses in four categories only: doing nothing, healing oneself, use of previously prescribed medicine and consulting a medical doctor. Only the four most common reactions are classified, and therefore the percentage does not sum up to 100.

seek external help and refuse the offer – by the medical establishment *and* by the alternative therapists – to consume a treatment or a therapy. Not even the marketing specialists concern themselves about those who decide *not* to consume treatment or therapy. They seem only to be concerned about consumers.

The Therapeutic Scene

One may wonder why nobody cares, and one may ask why the medical scientists do not concern themselves with fundamental issues about the consumption of treatments and about the kind of medical and therapeutic knowledge which is circulated in the alternative therapies; but conventional medical science is no longer competing with alternative medical knowledge, since science no longer struggles with the metaphysical distinction between truth and non-truth or between scientific truth and unscientific beliefs. Today, scientists have the belief, which is no doubt a metaphysical belief in disguise, that scientific discoveries are about finding correct technical solutions to a theoretical dispute.

A theoretical truth within medical science is disputed according to rules, standards and criteria which reproduce the scientific procedures – i.e., if the rules, standards and criteria are acceptable, it is a scientific result. Today, a scientific truth is what is accepted to be the truth at present within a concrete discipline which circulates medical knowledge in a network. The "ultimate" truth is what is produced and presented *now* according to accepted rules. This "ultimate" truth at present is a truth which is different from the truth which was produced, presented and circulated a few years back within the discipline. Transcended theories of the past are not claimed to be unscientific, since they have also followed the scientific procedures, but they are merely transcended by recent discoveries which are claimed to be the truth.

What I am suggesting is that we do not accept the competition between medical science and the alternative therapies as a matter of fact. It was certainly the case before (cf. Phillip Nicholls 1988, 1996), but today medical science does not struggle with alternative medical knowledge and practice, since medical science is competing within the networks of a concrete discipline or within the hierarchy of medical scientific periodicals.[4] I want to suggest that we see conventional, allopathic medicine which is legitimized by the knowledge of medical science,

---

4   Since 1945, the number of medical scientific periodicals has increased from 2,300 to 30,000, and today there are published more than 2 million medical scientific articles per year – i.e., 6,500 per day (cf. NASTRA 1995: 49).

and alternative therapies as two different therapeutic scenes which are not competing with each other.

Gerhard Schulze defines a scene as a subjective construction which many people adjust to each other (Schulze 1992: 472), and he argues that different scenes are not exclusive. A particular scene may be independent, but according to Schulze's study in Nürnberg in 1985, there is not an antagonistic relationship between hostile scenes. The relationships between the scenes are of affinity or of independence. They are not of an either-or structure, but rather of a both-and structure. We no longer find the kind of polarization which was the case before, between the scene of the aristocracy and the bourgeoisie and later between the scene of the bourgeoisie and the scene of the working class.

Today, polarization, aversion and intolerance are within the mind of the individual, and polarization goes in various directions, and aversion is directed toward various cultural distinctions by chance – i.e., intolerance is not in the relationship between the scenes; but in the mind of the individual.

What I am suggesting is that the polarization between conventional medicine and alternative medicine is in the mind of the individual, and that the aversion against allopathic medicine or against alternative therapies comes from various directions of the society and by chance, since aversion is in the mind of the individual, but aversion is constrained by the cultural repertoire of a lifestyle.

Gerhard Schulze's study in Nürnberg was intended to duplicate Pierre Bourdieus' famous study in France in the 1960s (Bourdieu 1979) which described a dynamic society where social and cultural distinctions are part of the struggle between the bourgeoisie, the petit bourgeoisie and the working class. The struggle for power in France in the 1960s was a matter of social practice and interactions in the economic and political life, within culture and in education, and Bourdieu's study demonstrated the correspondence between the social and cultural dimensions of modern societies.

Gerhard Schulze could not find such a correspondence between the cultural dimensions and the social dimensions in his material, but he found new tendencies, which were not described by Bourdieu, and which he called the Experience Society. Gerhard Schulze claims that we are experiencing a transformation between three scenarios which have caused the inner life of the individual (i.e., the subjectivity) to change. The first scenario is the reconstruction of the industrial society after 1945, the second has been described by Bourdieu, since it is the society of cultural conflicts and competition of the 1960s, and the third scenario is the contemporary experience society since the 1980s.

In our contemporary postmodern cultures, the subjectivity of the individual is no longer primarily concerned about producing goods in order to meet the needs of the individual, but the individual rather needs to choose what he or she wants.

And it is now a necessity that the individual decides what he or she wants *not* to choose, since the society is affluent, and the experience society offers an infinite number of choices. Gerhard Schulze suggests that modern man chooses among various experiences in order to experience that he lives. The individual in postmodern cultures makes choices in order to satisfy an internal need, which is both psychological and physical – i.e., a bodily defined need, which is internally motivated, and which is not necessarily defined by the external values and norms of the society.

I suggest as a hypothesis that the individual in postmodern cultures chooses to relate himself or herself to a therapeutic scene which offers a bodily experience which satisfies his or her internal need, and that the consumption of treatments and therapies relates the individual to a scene which adjusts the knowledge and practice of many people, since they share the same experience in the sense that they signify the scene by their consumption of treatment and therapy.

Gerhard Schulze has identified a number of different scenes in Nürnberg, and he describes six of them in his book; they are analyzed in relation to five major milieus: niveau-milieu, harmony-milieu, integration-milieu, selfrealization-milieu and entertainment-milieu, which are presented by Dirk Richter in this volume.[5] Schulze does not identify the scene of alternative therapies, and the reason is simply that his research instrument did not ask questions that would reveal the therapeutic scenes. Schulze's results have, however, twice been applied to socio-medical research in Germany by R. Jakob and U. Streeck (cf. Dirk Richter 1996). These studies reveal that a clear demand for alternative therapies can be predicted for the fourth milieu in Schulze's list – the self-realization-milieu.

Gerhard Schulze's study reveals that the self-realization-milieu is dominating in public and cultural life in Nürnberg, since it is closely related to the *Neue Kulturszene* (cf. note 5), which has become dominating for various reasons explained by Gerhard Schulze. This scene arose in the 1960s, and has become professionalized since the 1980s.

It is interesting for us to observe that the adherents of alternative therapies are recruited from the same milieu which is dominating in public and cultural life, since the scene which is intimately associated with the self-realization-milieu – i.e., *Neue Kulturszene* – is the dominating scene. The *Hochkulturszene*, which

---

5   The six scenes described by Gerhard Schulze are *Hochkulturszene, Neue Kulturszene, Kulturladenszene, Kneipenszene, Sportszene* and *Volksfestszene*. The second scene (i.e., the Neue Kulturszene) is characterized as: "*Kleinkunst, freie Theatergruppen, Jazz-Rock-Pop-Folk-Konzerte, Kabarett, Tanztheater, Filmkunst*" (Schulze 1992: 471).

attracts most members of the niveau-milieu since they associate themselves with this scene as a part of their lifestyle, and which is heavily funded by public money, is no longer the dominating scene; but the therapeutic scene, which is analogue with the *Hochkulturszene* in the sense that the niveau-milieu is attracted to it (i.e., to the hospitals and specialized clinics of allopathic medicine), and which is also heavily funded by public money, seems to be the dominating therapeutic scene in Denmark and in Germany.

Gerhard Schulze has not analyzed this complex situation, so we can only speculate about this observation. Perhaps the adherents of alternative therapies are dominating without knowing it, since they accept a representation of the situation which reproduces the concepts of the 1960s. These claim that the *Hochkulturszene* and the *Neue Kulturszene* are polarized, and repeat the idea that conventional medicine and alternative medical knowledge and practice are in conflict, since they compete for public funding, for privileges, for legitimacy and for prestige.

We can also only speculate about the complex situation observed earlier, that many Danes choose *not* to choose a treatment offered by conventional medicine *and* by alternative therapists. Since there is no information based on research on this cultural practice of non-doing, the floor is open for any kind of speculation, and all kinds of ideas can be projected upon the majority of the sick people who choose not to seek external help. One idea which is worth considering is that modern man has learned out of a necessity to make a choice, and that the individual in postmodern cultures to make the decision *not* to choose an offer which does not meet his internal needs, and which does not fit his lifestyle.

References

Andersen, J. Ø.
1992 "Sinhalese Buddhist Cosmology and Nature", in: O. Bruun & A. Kalland, (eds.): *Asian Perception of Nature*, Copenhagen.
1994 "Health Seeking in Pluralistic Health Care Systems", in: H. Johannessen, L. Launsø, S. Gosvig Olesen and F. Staugård, (eds.): *Studies in Alternative Therapies vol 1, Contributions from the Nordic Countries*, pp. 114-125, Odense University Press: Odense.
1995 "Alternativ Terapi og Betingelser for Viden", Centre for Cultural Research, Aarhus University.

Bourdieu, P.
1979 *La Distinction. Critique Sociale du Jugement*, Paris.

DIKE (Dansk Institut for Klinisk Epidemiologi)
1988 *Sundhed og sygelighed i Danmark, 1987*, Copenhagen.

Douglas, M.
1996 *Thought Styles*, London.

Institut for Fremtidsforskning
1994 *Den alment praktiserende læges patienter i de kommende 10 år*, Udarbejdet for ASTRA Danmark, Albertslund.

Johannessen, H.
1994 *Komplekse kroppe – alternativ behandling i antropologisk perspektiv*, Copenhagen.

Launsø, L.
1996a *Det alternative behandlingsområde. Brug og udvikling; rationalitet og paradigmer*, Copenhagen.
1996b "The Connection between Scope of Diagnosis and the User's Scope of Action – Empirical Findings and Theoretical Perspectives", (in this volume).

McQuire, M.
1988 *Ritual Healing in America*, New Brunswick and London.

NASTRA
1995 *Forslag til en national strategi for sundhedsvidenskab*, Forskningsministeriet, Copenhagen.

Nicholls, P. A.
1988 *Homoeopathy and the Medical Profession*, London.
1996 "A Hearing for Homoeopathy: Some Sociological Reflections on Problems of Communication about Alternative Therapy among Researchers and Practitioners" in: S. Gosvig Olesen and E. Høg (eds.): *Studies in Alternative Therapy 3. Communication in and about Alternative Therapies*, pp. 99-110, Odense University Press: Odense.

Richter, D.
1996 "Lifestyles – Different Cultural Pathways to Alternative Treatment", (in this volume).

Schulze, G.
1992 *Die Erlebnisgesellschaft. Kultursoziologie der Gegenwart*, Frankfurt/New York.

Lifestyles – Different Cultural Pathways to Alternative Treatment

by Dirk Richter

Conventional medicine has been controversially discussed for several decades. Different competing approaches have appeared to challenge medical expertise. At one time it was psychoanalysis, another time sociopolitical theories (Marxism etc.) which argued for discovering the blind spot of orthodox medicine. Now and then, alternative medical approaches have also appeared on the scene. In recent years, alternative approaches have seriously badgered the conventional medical practice. It is not my intention to justify this fact nor criticize it. The therapeutic successes of alternative medicine certainly deserve more attention from conventional medicine than they get today. At the same time, the theoretical foundations of alternative medicine are often questionable, if not dubious.

The aim of this paper is to attempt to find an answer to the question of the impact lifestyles of contemporary society have for the rise of alternative medical therapies and how these factors can be distinguished concerning different lifestyles we find today. My answer, however, will be a theoretical one. An empirical check of this matter is still to be taken.

Before regarding the critique that conventional medicine has to face these days, one has to remember that it is not the only institution being challenged now. Similar distrusting discourses can be found against politics, jurisdiction, public education, economy, and science. Politics is challenged because of numerous scandals and its inability to regulate the community. Jurisdiction is under attack because it cannot establish justice, only verdicts according to law. Public education is blamed for not teaching the norms that our society supposedly needs. Economy cannot any longer assure equal chances and opportunities for everybody. The problem with science is that it produces results which often have devastating consequences if they are implemented.

What all these criticizing verdicts have in common is that they reveal a deep mistrust toward our modern societal institutions. This is a rather new development in Western society. Looking back to the post-war era, especially to the 1950s, a large societal optimism was to be found. This optimism concerned nearly all social problems of that time, such as diseases, poverty or the overcoming of racial differences (Richter 1994a). And no doubt, this optimism could be found in theoretical analyses of the time as well as in everyday perception. Applying this description to the medical field, the years up to 1968 can be labelled *"The golden era of professional dominance"* (Pescosolido & Kronenfeld 1995: 13). The dominance of physicians within the medical field was unchallenged.

The first erosion of this positive atmosphere can be seen in the year 1968, when political uprising against traditional values and attitudes happened all over the Western world. From the end of the 1960s on, the distrust trickled out of the originally intellectual scene into the rest of society. Today, it affects nearly everybody in the Western hemisphere. The distrust against modern institutions has far-reaching consequences. As Anthony Giddens has shown, contemporary society is deeply based on trust (Giddens 1990). The transition from pre-modern social structure to modern society has led to the disembedding of social relations out of their local contexts, and their reconstruction across wide distances in time and space. Former face-to-face relations have been substituted by impersonal social contacts.

One of the significant elements of modernity Giddens identifies in this area is the development of expert systems. Societal expert systems (not expert systems in the sense of Artificial Intelligence) take over important functions such as expertise on building houses and bridges or expertise on curing diseases. We all more or less trust expert systems, often in a not-conscious manner. We do trust the bridges we are driving over, and we usually trust the diagnoses and treatment plans devised by our general practitioner. This trust in many expert systems provides the modern individual with an ontological security, and without this ontological security we could not lead a normal life (Giddens 1991).

Nevertheless, our usual trust in expert systems is more and more undermined, as discussed above. This deep and widespread distrust toward modern societal institutions I will call 'everyday postmodernism' in the following. Like the postmodernist attitude in social and philosophical theory which has questioned the 'grand narratives' of intellectual history (e.g., reason, progress), we find here a questioning of the 'grand institutions' which are still praised by political and other officials.

Conventional medicine underlies this everyday postmodernism, too. A UK poll from the early eighties showed that trust in orthodox medicine has diminished from 52% in 1978 to 39% in 1980 (cited by Fulder & Munro 1985). A further diminishing of trust in medicine in recent years can certainly be assumed. For many decades, official medicine has embodied the promise of curing severe diseases. While promising longevity it has concentrated mainly on acute illness and on pharmacological and surgical means. But, against all promises, we know

now that acute illness is only one problem among many others. Not only has orthodox medicine been unable to solve the problems of many acute diseases, it has lost sight of chronic diseases for several decades. The more or less exclusive focus on the named means of curing has made well-known traditional methods forgotten. The biomedical model, used as a dogma, turned out to be only one paradigm among others (Engel 1977). Although having thought to practice universally applicable methods, conventional medicine is now confronted with the realisation of having lost sight of important aspects of health and illness (Richter 1994b).

Furthermore, the one-sidedness of conventional medicine has led to an underestimation of normal living conditions. Think of the problems that large parts of oncology still have with prescribing opiates against severe pain even during the terminal phase. Or think of the reservations of many psychiatrists against polamidone treatment that allows the patient to lead an almost normal life on drugs. Only within the very last years has attention focused a little bit more on the meaning of illness in a patient's biography. The *"Illness Trajectory"*, as this topic has been called by Anselm Strauss and colleagues (Strauss *et al* 1985), is being realised more and more.

Those parts of life left unnoticed by conventional medicine, called 'Activities of Daily Living' are now the basis for nursing science. And along with nurses many other professions try to fill the gap not filled by medicine. As Pescosolido and Kronenfeld (1995: 16) have pointed out, today *"we are witnessing a renegotiation of the social contract of healing and the professional dominance of medicine (...) as well as the reemergence of alternative modes and thought and practice about health and illness"*.

The undergoing social change that has led to everyday postmodernism, however, is not only apparent in the skepticism against modern societal institutions. The social change affects the cultural system of society, too. As pointed out in detail below, the cultural sphere today is differentiated into several subcultural milieux. At this point, lifestyle appears on the scene. There is much theoretical as well as empirical evidence for describing the cultural sphere of Western society in terms of lifestyles. Lifestyles form the basis for the cultural self-understanding and self-interpretation of modern individuals.

Applied to the problem yet to be solved, the question emerges how do lifestyles influence the visiting behaviour of patients of alternative medical professions. My thesis is that we find different motivations within different lifestyles for visiting alternative therapies. Of course, it is a truism that there is not only one way to deal with matters of trust and distrust towards conventional medicine. Patients and clients of alternative treatments cannot be regarded as a homogeneous group (Schär, Messerli-Rohrbach & Schubarth 1994). In the following I will try to formulate a frame that can be used for a first theoretical answer to this question. To attempt to find this answer, I will take a short look at the concepts of lifestyle in sociological as well as in socio-medical research. After having compared these approaches, I will suggest relying on the 'social mileux'approach developed by Gerhard Schulze, that is applied to our question here. A short discussion will conclude this paper.

Lifestyle in Sociological Research

It is possibly not known within other scientific disciplines that the term "lifestyle" derives from sociological tradition. It may sound surprising, but the concept of "lifestyle" is nearly as old as sociology itself. Analysis of lifestyles belongs to sociological research almost from the beginning. Yet, at the startingpoint of sociology lifestyle was applied to investigate social inequality by theoretical means.

One of the first and most prominent lifestyle-theoreticians was Thorstein Veblen, who published his *"Theory of Leisure Class"* in 1899 (Veblen 1986). Veblen's research topic is the nonworking upper class. As the main feature of the leisure class, Veblen identifies the *conspicuous consumption*, i.e., the visibility and the symbolism of the conducted lifestyle. The wealth of these people had to be shown demonstratively. Veblen analyses, for example, the clothes as an expression of money.

Max Weber likewise belongs to the sociological lifestyle-research tradition. But: neither Veblen nor Weber used this term. Oddly enough, our usage of the term lifestyle derives from a slight translation error when Weber's *opus magnum* "*Economy and Society*" (Weber 1980) was translated into English (Abel 1991; Müller 1992). Weber used the words *"Lebensführung"* (life conduct) and *"Stilisierung des Lebens"* (stylization of life) which were taken together as "lifestyle" in the English and American editions. The retranslation has even led to the new word *"Lebensstil"* that did not exist before in the German language.

But from the philological problems back to sociological analysis: the topics Weber wanted to describe were the elements of the life conduct of the upper classes (Weber 1980: 537). The lifestyle-traits can be named, as in Veblen's investigation, as worklessness, many privileges, and a special sense of honour. Both, Veblen and Weber, noticed the function that those traits served as distinctive means against lower classes. Important is the symbolic quality that Weber and Veblen ascribed to the life conduct of the upper classes. In other words: from the beginning the expressive cultural dimension belongs to the sociological analysis of lifestyle.

The distinctive cultural elements of lifestyle remain the most important research topics, even after the Second World War. The French sociologist Pierre Bourdieu, to take one of the most important examples, investigates in his "Distinctions" the processes of social closure of lifestyles (Bourdieu 1982). With Bourdieu, still, lifestyles are related to economic inequality. The classes Bourdieu identifies as basic to modern social structure command different economic, social and cultural capital. But contrary to orthodox marxist class analysis, Bourdieu does not regard cultural expressions as determined by economic foundations. According to Bourdieu, lifestyles and matters of taste become a medium of symbolic class struggle apart from material struggles.

In recent years sociological research has postulated that lifestyles have even lost their close relations to classes and strata. By looking sharply at the 'new social inequality', it becomes clear that from the post-war years onwards the traditional classes and strata have vanished (although concepts of classes are still in use in social and medical research). Contemporarily, it is hardly possible to locate a person exclusively in one class or stratum. Think of the amount of workless academics that we face today all over Europe. To which class do they belong? Seen from an educational perspective they have to be placed in the highest stratum. The income of these persons, however, is often very poor. Today, we find a mixture of diverse cultural elements of different classes within one individual's life conduct. To refer to the cited example: the income may be low, but the consumed goods (e.g., books, films) may be those that have formerly been bought by the upper classes.

The social structure concerning inequality is more or less individualised. The concept of "risk society", developed by the German sociologist Ulrich Beck (1986), has gained a lot of attention in this regard. Risk society in the economic sense implies a notion of society as an elevator. You can get to the top very quickly, but the risk of falling down is very high. Compared with the previous decades, in the nineties an excellent education does not automatically lead to an excellent income. Specifically, risk society means to be left alone with all societal risks such as divorce and poverty.

But does the notion of an individualised risk society also imply that lifestyles have vanished, too? Empirical analyses, especially done by market research, reveal new patterns of consumption and new patterns of attitudes (Müller 1992). These new patterns no longer coincide exclusively with income or education. According to this research, new cultural clusters have been formed, and the items 'age' and 'education' are becoming the most important issues, whereas economic factors seem to be of minor importance. It seems that formerly unknown lifestyles have emerged. We are still beginning to learn the meaning of this message for the structure of Western society.

Lifestyle in Socio-medical Research

Regarded generally, it can observed that 'health' becomes more and more a super-value within contemporary Western society (Bauch 1996). Thus, a healthy lifestyle has become one of the most prominent topics in the contemporary way of living. Politicians, health insurance companies as well as advertising media call upon conducting one's life according to healthy rules.

In everyday reality, however, it is not so easy to follow these rules. This is the reason why 'lifestyle' has also become one of the most prominent terms in socio-medical research since the end of the 1960s. The concept of lifestyle in socio-medical research is likewise an answer to the fundamental change which Western society is undergoing. Thus, socio-economic stratification cannot be used as the main determinant for behavioural and attitudinal patterns.

The same can be said about the relation of class to health and illness. Classes or strata nowadays no longer have a direct impact on health and illness behaviour. Instead of classes and strata, one sees the lifestyle today as one of the most influential factors on individual health behaviour. Several epidemiological findings suggest that smoking, drinking or eating patterns cannot be attributed to socio-economic status exclusively. Still, economic indicators must not be underestimated in this question, but other features, such as living conditions, education, gender, or age also ought to be taken into account. These factors are important confounders when trying to predict illness occurrence and health behaviour.

But what is meant by the socio-medical use of lifestyle when examined in detail? Although it has been used now for several years as a basic assumption in medical theory as well as in empirical research, there is no clear, widely accepted definition. According to an official paper by the WHO Health Education Unit, lifestyle *"is taken to mean a general way of living based on the interplay between living conditions in the wide sense and individual patterns of behaviour as determined by sociocultural factors and personal characteristics"* (WHO Health Education Unit 1986: 118). Lifestyle is, in other words, a conglomeration of everything that plays a role in determining one's behaviour. Personal traits as well as environmental factors are to be considered.

This definition, of course, cannot be operationalised for empirical fieldwork. By reviewing the empirical literature on lifestyle in relation to health and illness affairs, it becomes clear that the concept of lifestyle is used here in a very restricted and limited way. What is usually examined is the health lifestyle a person conducts. Lifestyle is reduced to health-related behaviour and to attitudes towards health-related topics. In the literature you find questionnaires that ask for consumption patterns, attitudes concerning healthy living (such as 'worrying about getting sick'), or the person's appearance (Abel 1991). At the core of this lifestyle research stands the isolation of personality types which allow conclusions about consumption patterns and their means of prevention by goal-orientated influences (Troschke 1993). Thus, socio-medical lifestyle research aims at basics for developing prevention strategies by public health organisations.

From a methodological viewpoint the public health strategies according to socio-medical lifestyle research suggest that the health behaviour of a person is an option among many others. These strategies operate mostly by cognitive means, i.e., it is implicated that through a better knowledge about health risks, behaviour can basically be changed. In addition, there are attempts to offer alternative behavioural models. These models shall give the impression that there exist other ways of problem-solving than health-threatening habits. Even more, they suggest that the alternative models promise at least adequate satisfaction (Laaser, Hurrelmann & Wolters 1993). Such a strategy was chosen, for instance, by German public health institutions to demonstrate that as member of a sports-team you can experience as much joy as you feel when taking illicit drugs.

Lifestyle research in recent years has in this way contributed to a better understanding of the confounding factors of the onset of illness, and also to public health strategies against some of the most serious diseases (e.g., fitness strategies against coronary heart disease). The current research lacks, however, one fundamental notion related to lifestyle that we have seen in the sociological tradition. The cultural component that is acknowledged theoretically by socio-medical lifestyle research is more or less completely ignored. While aiming at the habits and the attitudes of individuals, the socio-cultural construction of habits and attitudes is pushed out of view.

Although the individualistic notion of lifestyle is backed by methodological premises as well as by psychological theory (Theory of Reasoned Action, Health Belief Model etc.), there is no clear indication that lifestyle is really an option to be chosen deliberately. Rather than the individualistic notion, it seems obvious to me that lifestyle patterns are deeply influenced by a person's social environment. For example, changing a peer group is one of the hardest efforts for adolescents. This reductionist use of lifestyle in current research has been criticised even within the field of lifestyle research (Backett & Davison 1995).

For this reason, the socio-medical lifestyle concept cannot be used to analyse the problem to be solved here. When asked for the identification of lifestyle elements for visiting alternative medical therapies the cultural, or even the subcultural, connotations of lifestyle have to be taken into account. Thus, returning to the sociological lifestyle concept seems unavoidable. In the following I will suggest use of a research approach which has received a lot of attention in recent years, at least within the German sociological discussion, as a starting-point for this project.

The Contemporary Western Society as 'Experience Society'

The fundamental social change of Western society has been mentioned several times. Looking at the structure of society, this change can be called an increasing differentiation of social systems. The social systems, such as politics, jurisdiction, education etc. work more and more self-referentially. These systems are steered exclusively from the inside. Today, we cannot identify a social system that steers the other systems in the sense of a superior one.

The ongoing differentiation of social systems, however, is only one side of society. On the other side, in everyday life, this differentiation of society finds its expression in the often cited "homeless mind" (Berger, Berger & Kellner 1973). The inability of one social system to take general responsibility for society is reflected by semantics of risk, uncertainty, and anxiety. The ontological security that Giddens has identified as basic for the functioning of modern life is vanishing more and more. We notice today "the end of unambiguity" as the subtitle of a book by Zygmunt Bauman (1991) indicates. Against all political, religious and other promises of certainty and orientation we experience ambivalence and contingency. This is the reason for the development of everyday postmodernism. Although orientation and security are claimed by the representatives of the social systems, we cannot trust them in the light of the more than obvious weaknesses that have been mentioned in the introduction. Regarding the culture of society as a whole, beyond all empirical differences that are dealt with in greater detail below, everyday postmodernism can be regarded as an integral part of the contemporary way of living.

However, this lack of orientation is unacceptable for most individuals. The search for new orientations, such as nationalism in politics or fundamentalism and New Age-ideas in the religious sphere, reflects obvious efforts to reduce ambivalence and contingency. And, by the way, it should be mentioned that many of the theoretical foundations of alternative medical therapies derive from these areas, too. One example is the topic of racism that has been found in the writings of Rudolf Steiner, the founder of Anthroposophy.

Apart from the cited social movements aiming at the reduction of individual uncertainty, we can find further collective patterns in everyday life. These patterns help to form new orientations 'below' those grand movements. It is the everyday aesthetics on which those patterns are based. Grounded on a large empirical investigation, the German sociologist Gerhard Schulze holds the thesis that, at least the German society, is structured by social milieux, providing the individual with such everyday aesthetics (Schulze 1992).

Schulze and his team found five major milieux in the second half of the 1980s in Germany: 1. niveau-milieu, 2. harmony-milieu, 3. integration-milieu, 4. self-realization-milieu, and 5. entertainment-milieu. What these milieux have in common is that they consist of internally shared collective notions of tokens, meanings, and knowledge. Yet, apart from all the differences in detail, those elements contribute to making 'experience' an all-embracing topic shared by all milieux. Regardless which milieu we analyse, we find, of course, different orientations focusing on making experiences. This is the reason why Schulze has chosen the title 'Experience Society' to label the contemporary cultural condition. In detail, of course, those named elements serve, as shown in the section above about sociological lifestyle research, as means to define distinction and similarity. Social milieux according to Schulze are on the whole similar to what has been called lifestyles in the sociological tradition.

What is covered by the milieu names of experience society? To start with *niveau-milieu*, it consists mainly of persons older than 40 years and with higher education. These people mainly work in educational professions, i.e., schools, universities etc. as well as in academic professions (as lawyer, physician etc.). Their entertainment preferences are as follows: visiting concerts, listening to classical music, reading books, being interested in politics, culture, economy and history. The distinction patterns can be named as anti-barbaric, no trivial literature, no watching of quiz-shows and other TV-programs. The primary perspective of the niveau-milieu is hierarchical; striving for high ranks in society is existential.

The persons in *harmony-milieu* are also older than 40 years, but have only lower education. They typically earn their money as workers and saleswomen. Often they are pensioners. Harmony-milieu mainly prefers what is avoided by niveau-milieu, namely TV-shows, German pop songs, pulp fiction and so on. The distinction patterns are classical and rock music, quality newspapers and so on. When the persons in harmony-milieu enjoy something, it has to do with snugness. Their primary perspective is sensing danger, and thus they strive for security.

Persons who are described as belonging to *integration-milieu* are usually older than 40 years, too, and they have middle education. They work mainly as middle employees and civil servants. The preference patterns cannot be identified as clearly as in the other milieux. The label 'integration' stands for preference patterns for high culture as well as for the minor educated milieux. The distinction patterns are anti-eccentric and anti-barbaric, too. This milieu existentially strives for conformity and normality.

Self-realization-milieu consists of persons under 40 years, coupled with middle or higher education. The professions of this milieu are often social, therapeutical and educational jobs. These persons like going out to festivals, they visit pubs, and they spend a lot of money travelling. They are often intellectually orientated and read quality papers. Persons in the self-realization-milieu dissociate themselves from trivial orientation. As indicated by the label, they strive for self-realization; spontaneity is a fundamental part of their lives.

The last milieu, named *entertainment-milieu*, consists of younger people under 40 years with a low level of education. They earn their living as younger workers and salespeople. Persons of the entertainment-milieu are often football-fans and visit bodybuilding-studios and game halls. They like driving cars or motorcycles and they spend large sums for their maintenance. The distinction patterns that can be named are high culture, classical music and theatre as well as quality papers. The existential orientation of this milieu is striving for stimulation. One's own needs stand in the centre of orientation.

It should be mentioned, of course, that these milieux have to be seen as idealtypical; i.e., the milieux serve mainly as analytical orientations. In reality, the elements are not often found together.

Lifestyles – Shaping the Pathway to Alternative Therapies

The introduction of the social milieux according to Schulze should have made clear that modern lifestyles include a cultural orientation. By providing subcultural attitudes, values and even distinction patterns, lifestyles help the individual to get oriented within the confusing conditions of modernity. The orientation gap left by politics is basically filled by subcultural lifestyles. This statement is also valid for the orientation within the field of medical therapies. I hold the thesis that modern lifestyles fundamentally shape the access to alternative medical therapies. In this section the thesis is worked out in detail.

Although the thesis remains theoretical it can be supported by further empirical findings. Schulze's results have twice been applied to topics of sociomedical research. One study, done by sociologists of the university of Trier, Germany, has analysed the impact of social milieux on the perception of illness, especially on the perception of AIDS (Jacob 1995). Their findings support Schulze's results in general. On a continuum, with harmony-milieu on one side and self-realization-milieu on the other side, the perceptions and attitudes against AIDS could be located. Whereas the harmony-milieu had the least knowledge of HIV-infected persons and the greatest fear against AIDS, in self-realization-milieu quite the opposite was found. The fear of carriers of the HI-virus was very low for younger persons with higher education living mostly in urban areas. The antithetical traits of the harmony- and self-realization-milieux has also been noticed by Schulze (Schulze 1992: 312).

A second study, done by psychiatrists of the Niedersächsisches Landeskrankenhaus Rosdorf-Tiefenbrunn, Germany, analysed the milieu-background of their patients in ambulant psychotherapy (Streeck 1993). This study also supported Schulze's findings, showing divergent patterns of attitudes toward psychotherapy and different patterns of visiting behaviour among the social milieux. Persons located in the niveau-milieu asked mostly for psychoanalysis as therapeutical method. In contrast, persons from harmony-milieu reacted to self-reflective forms of psychotherapy mostly with a lack of understanding and perplexity. Persons located within the self-realization-milieu have had mostly a lot of experience with several different therapeutical methods before visiting the hospital. Many people of self-realization-milieu have contact with what is called the 'psycho-scene' in Germany.

The results of the cited studies show an immense impact of lifestyle or subcultural milieu on attitudes and behaviour related to health, illness and therapy. What conclusions for the visiting behaviour of alternative medical therapies among the different milieux can be drawn from these findings?

It seems evident to me to assume a divergent visiting behaviour similar to that shown by the study on psychotherapy. For niveau-milieu it can be supposed that conventional medicine still remains the valid paradigm. Everyday postmodernism is least distinctive within this group compared to the other milieux. Due to the academic education of niveau-milieu, alternative therapies cannot so easily be communicated. Alternative therapies find most acceptance when they are applied by physicians or other persons with an academic education or with a scientific background. The mode of effectiveness of the therapy must be comprehensible. This way, the risk of being a subject of 'quackery' is minimised. Clearly, the locus of control of the individuals in this group is internal. The integration of alternative therapies into conventional medicine that can be observed today makes the access to alternative therapies easier for this group.

The visiting behaviour of harmony-milieu cannot be predicted as easily. One of the most important traits of harmony-milieu is, though seldom communicated, general distrust. Thus, on one side, alternative therapies, usually not known within the everyday life of this group, are reacted to with the same lack of understanding found in the study on psychotherapy. Schulze (1992) as well as Jacobs (1995) found in their studies high rates of fatalism within harmony-milieu. Persons from harmony-milieu mainly construct their locus of control externally. For this reason, changing the therapy, i.e., actively leaving conventional medicine, seems rather unlikely for this group. On the other side, one observes that alternative therapies gain access to this milieu in other ways. At least in Germany, the tabloid press, which is read mainly by this milieu, reports a lot on alternative approaches in medicine. Of course, the aim of those reports is not factual information for their readers. Rather than objective information it can be labelled as sensation-seeking in the sense of 'A New Wonder Therapy'. Nevertheless, doubt about conventional medicine is communicated in each such report. Changing to alternative approaches is more likely when conventional medicine fails completely, especially when patients suffer from chronic illnesses. In this case, the fatalism described above is likewise shown towards alternative therapies. In contrast to niveau-milieu, the mode of effectiveness need not be comprehended in harmony-milieu.

As Schulze has found, normality and conformity are leading values for integration-milieu. Many alternative therapies have lost their notion of unconventionality in recent years. Thus, visiting such a therapy would not be ruled out by persons of this group. But, conventional medicine still remains the 'normal' paradigm for integration-milieu. Concerning fatalism this milieu holds a medium position. It shows more fatalism than self-realization-milieu, but less than harmony-milieu. On the whole, alternative therapies are accepted, but within integration-milieu they are not often asked for.

In contrast to all other milieux, a more than clear demand for alternative curing methods can be predicted for self-realization-milieu. As indicated by further empirical research on this topic, clients of alternative methods are mainly highly educated, aged under 50, and female (Moore *et al* 1985; Fulder & Munro 1985; Schär, Messerli-Rohrbach & Schubarth 1994). Even Schulze found in his study for this group an orientation towards discovering and curing the 'inner self' (Schulze 1992: 314, 318). Meditation, yoga, dancing therapy as well as different forms of psychotherapy (e.g., sensitivity groups) belong to the accepted methods of curing oneself. Within this group the locus of control is clearly internal; fatalism is to be found least among all milieux. Changing therapies (and therapists) happens very often. The way of gaining information about alternative medical methods is related to the internal locus of control. We find an active search for knowledge about those methods mostly from the many and diverse books on counselling. Thus, acceptance of new and formerly unknown methods is larger than among the other milieux. Additionally, the theoreticians of New Age (e.g., Capra, Ferguson) are read more or less exclusively by this milieu. In this way, the everyday postmodernism of self-realization-milieu gets its theoretical foundation. By reflecting actively on the different approaches and their supposed theoretical background (holism, cultural contexts etc.) one assumes to comprehend the modes of effectiveness. Self-realization-milieu is the only milieu where active reflection on those methods is to be found. These assumptions are supported by empirical studies which found strong post-materialistic and holistic attitudes among patients of alternative treatments (Schär, Messerli-Rohrbach & Schubarth 1994).

Persons from the last milieu, entertainment-milieu, are least likely to visit alternative therapies. This group mainly sticks to conventional medicine; it does not visit psychotherapy either (Streeck 1993). Similar to harmony-milieu, distrust, fatalism and rigidity are important traits of thinking, but these traits are less distinctive than in harmony-milieu. "Doctor knows best" is the motto of the entertainment-milieu.

Conclusion

The aim of this paper has been to find out which impact lifestyles of contemporary society have on the visiting behaviour for alternative medical therapies. The widespread critique against conventional medicine is regarded as part of everyday postmodernism, an attitude that has affected most members of Western society. Everyday postmodernism expresses a deep distrust toward most of the modern societal institutions. Among members of Western society the postmodernist attitudes towards conventional medicine are articulated in different ways.

It has been suggested that the social-milieu concept of Gerhard Schulze could be used to analyse in detail the differences between the lifestyles. The social-milieu concept derives from sociological lifestyle research tradition. Compared to the use of lifestyle in socio-medical research, the original sociological lifestyle-concept has the advantage of referring to the cultural background of Western society and its differentiations.

It could be shown theoretically that social milieux have a deep impact on attitudes towards health, illness and visiting behaviour for alternative medical therapies. Everyday postmodernism related to the medical field, and thus to the different visiting behaviour for alternative therapies, is fundamentally shaped by the subcultural notions of the milieux.

The relevance of lifestyles for therapeutical praxis and the effectiveness of the different methods also becomes evident. A better knowledge about the milieu-background of patients and clients could possibly lead to a better compliance. One important feature, influenced by lifestyle, is the notion of the patient's own contribution in regaining health. Active participation in curing oneself on the part of the patient cannot be ignored by alternative therapists, nor by conventional physicians. For alternative methods, too, the *"work of patients"* (Strauss *et al* 1985), as a contribution to one's own health, must certainly deserve more attention. This aspect was recently emphasized by a study on the impact of the patient's expectations on the effectiveness of alternative therapies (Wirth 1995).

May a last open question be permitted to the sociologist author of this paper. Many alternative therapies (e.g., classical homeopathy) work on the assumption that illness symptoms are closely related to the personality traits of the patient. In my opinion, one should ask how large the contributing part of personality really is and which part is played by the patient's socio-cultural context. The great impact of lifestyles and milieux on attitudes and behaviour related to health and illness indicated in this paper could also have implications for these methodological questions of alternative therapies.

References

Abel, Thomas
1991 "Measuring Health Lifestyles in a Comparative Analysis: Theoretical Issues and Empirical Findings", in: *Social Science and Medicine*, 32: 899-908.

Backett, Kathryn C., Charlie Davison
1995 "Lifecourse and Lifestyle: The Social and Cultural Location of Health Behaviours", in: *Social Science and Medicine*, 40: 629-638.

Bauch, Jost
1996 *Gesundheit als sozialer Code. Von der Vergesellschaftung des Gesundheitswesens zur Medikalisierung der Gesellschaft,* Juventa: Weinheim/München.

Bauman, Zygmunt
1991 *Modernity and Ambivalence,* Polity Press: Oxford.

Beck, Ulrich
1986 *Risikogesellschaft. Auf dem Weg in eine andere Moderne*, Suhrkamp: Frankfurt/M.

Berger, Peter L., Brigitte Berger, Hansfried Kellner
1973 *The Homeless Mind. Modernization and Consciousness,* Random House: New York.

Bourdieu, Pierre
1982 *Die feinen Unterschiede,* Suhrkamp: Frankfurt/M.

Engel, George L.
1977 "The Need for a New Medical Model: A Challenge for Biomedicine", in: *Science*, 196: 129-136.

Fulder, St.J., R.E. Munro
1985 "Complementary Medicine in the United Kingdom: Patients, Practitioners, and Consultations", in: *Lancet*, II: 542-545.

Giddens, Anthony
1990 *The Consequences of Modernity*, Stanford University Press: Stanford, Ca.
1991 *Modernity and Self-Identity: Self and Society in the Late Modern Age,* Polity Press: Cambridge, England.

Jacob, Reiner
1995   *Krankheitsbilder und Deutungsmuster. Wissen über Krankheit und dessen Bedeutung für die Praxis,* Westdeutscher Verlag: Opladen.

Laaser, Ulrich, Klaus Hurrelmann, Paul Wolters
1993   "Prävention, Gesundheitsförderung und Gesundheitserziehung", in: Hurrelmann, Klaus and Laaser, Ulrich (eds.): *Gesundheitswissenschaften. Handbuch für Lehre, Forschung und Praxis,* pp. 176-203, Beltz: Weinheim.

Moore, J., K. Phipps, D. Marcer, G. Lewitt
1985   "Why do People Seek Treatment by Alternative Medicine?", in: *British Medical Journal,* 290: 28-29.

Müller, Hans-Peter
1992   *Sozialstruktur und Lebensstile. Der neuere theoretische Diskurs über soziale Ungleichheit,* Suhrkamp: Frankfurt/M.

Pescosolido, Bernice A., Janice J. Kronenfeld
1995   "Health, Illness, and Healing in an Uncertain Era: Challenges from and for Medical Sociology", in: *Journal of Health and Social Behavior,* Extra Issue: 5-33.

Richter, Dirk
1994a   "Der Mythos der 'guten' Nation. Zum theoriegeschichtlichen Hintergrund eines folgenschweren Mißverständnisses", in: *Soziale Welt,* 45: 304-321.
1994b   "Existentialism and Postmodernism. Continuities, Breaks, and some Consequences for Medical Theory", in: *Theoretical Medicine,* 15: 253-265.

Schär, A., V. Messerli-Rohrbach, P. Schubarth.
1994   "Schulmedizin oder Komplementärmedizin: Nach welchen Kriterien entscheiden sich die Patientinnen und Patienten?", in: *Schweizerische Medizinische Wochenschrift,* 124 (Suppl. 62): 18-27.

Schulze, Gerhard
1992   *Die Erlebnisgesellschaft. Kultursoziologie der Gegenwart,* Campus: Frankfurt/M./New York.

Strauss, Anselm, Shizuko Fagerhaugh, Barbara Suczek, Carolyn Wiener
1985   *Social Organization of Medical Work,* University of Chicago Press: Chicago/London.

Streeck, Ulrich
1993   "Psychotherapie und soziale Milieus", in: *Psychologische Beiträge,* 35: 76-86.

Troschke, Jürgen von
1993   "Gesundheits- und Krankheitsverhalten", in: Hurrelmann, Klaus and Laaser, Ulrich (eds.): *Gesundheitswissenschaften. Handbuch für Lehre, Forschung und Praxis,* pp. 155-175, Beltz: Weinheim.

Veblen, Thorstein
1986   *Theorie der feinen Leute. Eine ökonomische Untersuchung der Institutionen,* Fischer: Frankfurt/M. (orig. 1899).

Weber, Max
1980   *Wirtschaft und Gesellschaft. Grundriss der verstehenden Soziologie,* 5th ed., Mohr: Tuebingen (orig. 1922).

WHO Health Education Unit
   1986   "Life-Styles and Health", in: *Social Science and Medicine*, 22: 117-124.

Wirth, Daniel P.
   1995   "The Significance of Belief and Expectancy within the Spiritual Healing Encounter", in: *Social Science and Medicine*, 41: 249-260.

Lifestyle, Beliefs and Value Systems, and Complementary Medicine

by Adrian Furnham

To what extent is an interest in, knowledge about, or preference for, Complementary Medicine (CM) simply a product of lifestyle? Or is CM intimately bound up with belief or value systems? That is, do people become involved with CM because the apparent values of CM practices, as they understand them, fit in with or reflect their values? Has an increase in interest about CM come about because of the growth of the green movement, post-materialists cults, or new age philosophy? This chapter addresses these issues with special reference to the concept of lifestyle and psychological analysis.

The Concept of Lifestyle

The term lifestyle is used in many contexts and has come to denote many things. It has usually been used to denote general conditions of living which entail an element of personal action at the individual level. Within the health and medical context, lifestyle is usually covered by topics such as diet, leisure/exercise activities, intake of drugs (including alcohol and tobacco), personal body maintenance (hygiene, sleep) as well as reactions to stress. Davison *et al* (1992) argue that one should limit the term *"to those behaviours and conditions which official and commercial health promotion has strongly associated with the possibility of individual choice and the triumph of self-control over self-indulgence"* (Davison et al 1992: 675).

They note that there are aspects of life which affect health but are clearly not part of lifestyle. These include differences in heredity and upbringing; differences in the social and physical environment; and the operation of chance and luck. Thus, whilst these factors are beyond one's control, lifestyle is supposedly something over which one does have control.

The concern of many in both orthodox and complementary medicine is that many people do not comply with "healthy lifestyle" advice. Non-compliance has been attributed to ignorance and lack of knowledge. It has also been attributed to the apparently widespread fatalistic belief that health is largely determined by forces outside the control of the individual. Certainly, lay notions of luck, fate, destiny, randomness and chaos are strongly associated with health.

Backett and Davison (1995) argue: *"At its most basic in health research, lifestyle may be seen as a behaviour or set of behaviours which are typical for an individual or group"* (Backett & Davison 1995: 630). They further note that *"in classical theory, therefore, lifestyle denotes an inter-related pattern of conduct for the individual, an expression of belonging to a particular group, and some suggestion of structural life chances"* (ibid.: 631). More modern writers see lifestyle as adopted or chosen (a cluster of habits and orientations) rather than 'handed down', forced to accept or inherited. Certainly life chances condition lifestyle choices.

The concept of lifestyle has been attractive to CM practitioners, because it has holistic and ecological overtones, and seems to allow for the often tangled and complex relationships between social, cultural, political and economic forces. Yet the term remains vague. For marketeers, the term is used to refer to the consumption and behaviour patterns of different social groups. For health researchers, it has come to describe and categorize the differences in beliefs and practices between groups in the population.

> "Here lifestyle provides the ill defined link (or 'target') between epidemiologically designated health risk factors at the individual level (notably drinking, smoking, diet, substance abuse, levels of exercise, and latterly, unprotected sexual intercourse) and preventive medicine or health promotion at the population level. In many such applications, lifestyle has therefore been used to draw together some combination of discrete behaviours with little reference to the social and cultural contexts in which they are embedded and given meaning" (Backett & Davison 1995: 631).

Ordinary lay people use the term lifestyle even more vaguely and loosely. They nearly always confuse the socio-physical conditions within which they live and the things they do within them. For many it is the daily routines and activities in response to environmental givens. That is, it involves both the quality and the mode of life. Further, lay people see lifestyle as a set of culturally acceptable behaviours that are appropriate for a person depending on age, class, and personal history.

Psychographics, Lifestyle and Complementary Medicine

Psychographics is the principal technique used by consumer researchers as a measure of lifestyle analysis. One aim of psychographics is to provide quantitative measures of consumer lifestyles, while another is to understand the complex pattern of potential and consumer's lives (Cathelat 1993). The collection and analysis of exclusively demographic data (e.g., sex, age, class) are often not sufficient aids in the planning of marketing programs because demographics do not answer many questions. A selected list of these questions asked by psychographics researchers are:

- "Why do consumers act as they do?"
- "Why do consumers with similar demographic characteristics act differently?"
- "Why do consumers become brand loyal or regularly switch brands?"
- "Why do some consumers act as innovators and buy products before others?"
- "Under what situations do families employ joint decision making?"
- "How do consumers behave when shopping for a product?"
- "Why does status play a large role in the purchase of some goods and a small role in the purchase of others?"
- "How does risk affect consumer decisions?"
- "How do motives affect consumer decisions?"
- "How important is a purchase decision to a consumer?"
- "How long will it take for a consumer to reach a purchase decision?"
- "To whom does a consumer look for advice prior to purchasing?"

In an attempt to answer these and other questions, marketers, in increasing numbers, are using demographic data in conjunction with, and as part of, social, psychological, and consumer decision-making analysis. For those social and psychological factors from a marketing perspective comprise a consumer's *lifestyle*, which is the pattern in which a person lives and spends time and money. A lifestyle combines the influences of personality and social values that have been internalized by an individual. A person's demographic background has a strong influence on the lifestyle, or way of living, adopted. Lifestyles are the result of the total array of economic, cultural, social life forces that contribute to a person's human qualities. Most directly, lifestyle is a derivative of the social values a person internalizes and an individual's personality.

The concept of lifestyle is built upon the social-psychological theory that people develop constructs with which to interpret, predict, and control their environment. These constructs or patterns result in behaviour patterns and attitude structures maintained to minimize incompatibilities and inconsistencies in a person's life—thus, it is possible to measure patterns, called lifestyles, among groups of people. Psychographics or AIO measures are the operational form of lifestyles which marketing researchers measure. AIO stands for Activities, Interests, and Opinions, and may be either general or product-specific.

The concept and name of psychographics were originated by Demby (1974) to describe a technique that added the richness of the social and behavioural sciences to demographics. Demby provided a three-level definition of psychographics:

1. Behavioural and social sciences applied to marketing research.
2. More specifically, psychographics is a quantitative research procedure that is indicated when demographic, socioeconomic, and user/non-user analyses are not sufficient to explain and predict consumer behaviour.
3. Most specifically, psychographics seeks to describe the human characteristics of consumers that may have bearing on their response to products, packaging, advertising and public relations efforts. Such variables may span a spectrum from self-concept and lifestyle to attitudes, interests and opinions, as well as perceptions of product attributes.

There has been some dispute between marketing practitioners and academic researchers as to what constitutes psychographics — and whether or not it is synonymous with lifestyle research. The consensus appears to be that there is a distinction between the two concepts. Psychographics refers to customers' personality traits (e.g., their sociability, self-reliance, assertiveness, etc.), while lifestyles consist primarily of individual's Activities, Interests and Opinions (or AIOs). Some researchers use the A to stand for attitudes, but activities are a better measure of lifestyles because they measure what people do. AIO components are defined by Reynolds and Darden (1974) as follows:

> "An activity is a manifest action such as viewing a medium, shopping in a store, or telling a neighbour about a new service. Although these acts are usually observable, the reasons for the actions are seldom subject to direct measurement. An interest in some object, event or topic is the degree of excitement that accompanies both special and continuing attention of it. An opinion is a verbal or written 'answer' that a person gives in response to a stimulus situation in which some 'question' is raised. It is used to describe interpretations, expectations, and evaluations – such as beliefs about the intentions of other people, anticipations concerning future events, and appraisals of the rewarding or punishing consequences of alternative courses of action."

Examples of each AIO category are shown in Table 1. Demographics are also undivided in most studies involving such variables.

Table 1: AIO categories of lifestyle studies

ACTIVITIES	INTERESTS	OPINIONS	DEMOGRAPHICS
Work	Family	Themselves	Age
Hobbies	Home	Social issues	Education
Social events	Job	Politics	Income
Vacation	Community	Business	Occupation
Entertainment	Recreation	Economics	Family size
Club membership	Fashion	Education	Dwelling
Community	Food	Products	Geography
Shopping	Media	Future	City size
Sports	Achievements	Culture	Stage in lifestyle

Source: Plummer, Joseph T. (1974).

It is indeed possible that health issues appear in each column, particularly interests and opinions. The specific approach to AIOs focuses on statements that are product-specific and that identify benefits associated with the product or brand. For instance, one study concerned with health-care services included both general and specific statements (Blackwell & Talarzyk 1977). The study was concerned with predicting what types of consumers try to behave in a way that will achieve consistency between their behaviour and attitudes. It was necessary to determine specific attitudes toward physicians as well as toward malpractice. Thus, statements such as the following were included:

1. I have a great deal of confidence in my own doctor.
2. About half of the physicians are not really competent to practice medicine.
3. Most physicians are overpaid.
4. In most malpractice suits, the physician is not really to blame.

In this study, respondents who indicated that they have a great deal of confidence in their doctors, also reported a much lower likelihood of bringing a malpractice suit. Respondents agreeing with statements that physicians are not really competent and that they are overpaid, disagreed with the statements that physicians are not really to blame in malpractice suits, and were more likely to file a malpractice suit. Also those who agreed with general AIO statements, such as "I generally do exercises" and "I am sick a lot more than my friends are", were found to be more likely to bring malpractice suits.

In another much more typical psychographic study, the purpose of which was to explore relationships between consumers' lifestyle and their overall product-assortment decisions, Cosmas (1982) used a postal questionnaire containing 250 AIO items and 179 frequency-of-use items. A technique called Q-factor analysis was used to compute lifestyle and product topologies. The lifestyle clusters generated were: (1) Traditionalist, (2) Frustrated, (3) Life-Expansionists, (4) Mobiles, (5) Sophisticates, (6) Actives, and (7) Immediate Gratifiers. The product clusters were: (1) Personal Care, (2) Shelf-Stocker, (3) Cooking and Baking, (4) Self-Indulgent, (5) Social, (6) Children's, and (7) Personal Appearance. In addition to the above tests, an 'eyeballing' of the data suggested the relationships described below. This, in turn, seemed to reflect the Traditionalists' way of life, which placed emphasis on the role of women as homemakers. The relationships were defined thus:

Frustrated

The *Frustrateds'* product-assortment decision tended to be weak on the Social dimension and unrelated to any of the others. This indicated that Frustrateds tend to be unsure about what they like and unable to find satisfaction in product purchase in any clearly defined way.

Life-Expansionist

The *Life-Expansionists'* product-assortment tendencies were characterised by weak dispositions towards Shelf Stocking, Self-Indulgence, and Personal Appearance. This reflect the Life-Expansionists' way of life which places emphasis on involvement with their environment and a rejection of self-centredness.

Mobile

The *Mobiles'* product-related behaviours were characterised by strong Self-Indulgence, Children's and Personal Appearance tendencies. The Mobiles' way of life placed emphasis on careful eating habits, and more emphasis on themselves and other members of the family, due to a lack of social ties.

Active

The *Actives'* product-related attributes were characterised by Personal Care, Self-Indulgence, and Personal Appearance factors. This reflects the Actives' way of life which placed emphasis on meeting people, going places, and just being on the go.

Sophisticated

The *Sophisticateds'* product-related characteristics were defined by Personal

Care and Social product dimensions. Sophisticates tended to place emphasis on the social and external events in their environment.

Immediate Gratifiers
Finally, the *Immediate Gratifiers* were characterised by Personal Care, Cooking and Baking, Self-Indulgence and Social factors. The Immediate Gratifiers desire instant satisfaction and crave hedonistic activities.

This is the typical typology that results from a psychographic analysis. Once that has been established, the specific health related behaviours (i.e., consumption of vitamins, purchasing of skin creams; interest in aromatherapy oils) are considered within each category.

The Basic Values System

There have been several attempts to produce psychological typologies of lifestyle which can cover the entire active consumer population. These studies have generated psychographic segmentations which comprise basic categories of consumers defined in terms of their reported values and lifestyles. These systems are purported to yield enduring psychological constructs which define the broadest consumer populations, but which also predict idiosyncratic behaviour.

One of the most widely popularised approaches to lifestyle research for market segmentation on this scale is the VALS (Values and Lifestyles) programme developed by Mitchell (1983) in California. It started from the theoretical base of Maslow's need hierarchy and the concept of social character (Riesman, Glazer & Denney 1950). The essence of the VALS programme is a classification scheme that assigns people to one of nine VALS segments. These segments are determined by *both* the values and lifestyles of the people in them. "Values" within this system refers to a wide array of an individual's beliefs, hopes, desires, aspirations, prejudices and so on. Conceptually, VALS represents a linkage between the personality orientation of psychographics and the activities orientation of lifestyle research. The "nine American lifestyles" defined in this programme, together with typical demographics and buying patterns, are shown in Table 2.

The basic belief behind VALS is that humans strive to improve themselves during their lifetime, which strongly influences their values, lifestyles and many of the decisions they make each day. The approach is holistic, drawing on insight from a number of perspectives and many types of data to develop a comprehensive framework of characterising the ways of life of Americans.

The core of the VALS programme is the VALS typology or current day lifestyles. This typology is hierarchial. The VALS system defines a typology of four basic categories of consumer values and lifestyles, with nine more detailed types. Drawing originally from Maslow, SRI International describes consumer market segments as *Need-Driven, Outer-Directed, Inner-Directed*, and *Integrated*. The argument is that there are basic needs which have to be satisfied to survive and sustain existence. With affluence Need-Driven motives give way to expression of the sort of person you are, following pathways of earlier Outer-Direction or Inner-Direction through ways of living, products bought, and so on.

The prime developmental thrust is from Need-Driven through Outer-Directed and Inner-Directed phases, to a journey of Outer and Inner-Directions. These major transitions are seen as crucial stage posts in the movement of an individual (or a society) from immaturity to full maturity (psychological maturity). Very generally, psychological maturation is marked by a progression from partial toward full realization of one's potential. It involves a steady widening of perspectives and concerns, and a steady deepening of the inner influence points consulted in making important decisions.

The VALS topology is divided into four major categories, within each of which there are several segments (except the Integrateds, which is so small that it is a segment in itself). These lifestyle segments are fitted together into what is called the VALS double hierarchy. In total, there are nine VALS segments, with every adult theoretically fitting into one of these categories. Table 2 summarizes some of the demographic characteristics of these segments.

The lifestyle groups in the United States include survivors (4 per cent), sustainers (7 per cent), belongers (37 per cent), emulators (8 per cent), achievers (22 per cent), I-am-me's (3 per cent), experiential (6 per cent), societally-conscious (11 per cent), and integrated (2 per cent). A proprietary system of weighting questions for classification was developed using data from a national probability of 1,635 Americans and their spouses/mates (1078) who responded to an SRI International mail survey in 1980. VALS has had considerable impact since that time. Part of its allure comes from the vivid individual portraits that advocates paint of members of the various groups.

Need-Driven consumers exhibit spending by need rather than preference, and are subdivided into survivors and sustainers, the former among the most disadvantaged people in the economy. Outer-Directed consumers, who are divided into three sub-groups, are the backbone of the marketplace, and generally buy with awareness of what other people will attribute to their consumption of that product. Inter-Directed consumers are divided into three subgroups. They comprise a much smaller percentage of the population. Their lives are directed more toward their individual needs than toward values orientated to externals.

Although their numbers are small, they may be important as trend setters or groups through which successful ideas and products trickle up. This segment is growing rapidly, whereas the number of Need-Driven consumers is declining and Outer-Directed is holding steady.

Table 2: Key demographics of the VALS segments

		AGE (median)	SEX (% female)	RACE (% white)	EDUCATION (years)	INCOME (household)
I.	**Need Driven**					
	Survivors	66[a]	60%	55%	8.5	$5,000
	Sustainers	32	52	67	10.0	9,000
II.	**Outer-Directed**					
	Belongers	54	60	92	11.0	14,000
	Emulators	28	48	76	12.5	19,000
	Achievers	42	39	95	13.5	35,000
III.	**Inner-Directed**					
	I-Am-Me's	20	42	87	11.5	12,500
	Experientials	26	61	96	14.0	26,000
	Societally Conscious	38	54	89	15.0	30,000
IV.	**Integrateds**	40	54	93	16.0	34,000

[a] Age is expressed as median years, education as mean years completed, and income as median 1980 dollars per household in each segment.

Source: SRI International, VALS – *Values and Lifestyles of Americans* (Menlo Park, Calif.: SRI International, undated), p.4.

It may be worth speculating, within each segment, about how each type would react to complementary medicine (CM).

The "Need-Driven" Lifestyle (11% of the population)
These people's values and lifestyles are very strongly affected by restrictions in money available to them. Their values tend to centre on the immediate and to focus on safety, security, and survival. As consumers, these people buy more from need than by choice and desire. Within this type, there are two specific market segments — Survivors and Sustainers.

"Survivors" are the very bottom of the hierarchy. This segment accounts for about 4% of all adults. They are the most disadvantaged of people because of their age (average age is about 66 years), lower levels of education and income, and lack of prospects for life to get much better in the future. Many of the people in this segment lived most of their lives at higher levels of the VALS hierarchy, but now face a combination of economic and health problems that dominate their lives. The values of this group are traditional in nature. Minorities are over-represented in this group, as are women, due to longer life expectancies. It is unlikely that this group is very interested in CM except in that they may be reliant on one particular method they have access to (i.e., chiropractice). On the other hand, they may be fairly enthusiastic about some (cheap) CM methods, precisely because they cannot afford orthodox medicine. Thus, they are most likely to be drawn to CM not because of ideology but because they could not afford or get satisfaction from orthodox medicine.

"Sustainers" account for 7% of the population. These people are much younger (average age 32) than the Survivor segment, but they also face economic restrictions that have a strong impact on their lives. This group also has low levels of education, and minorities are again over-represented. This group is at the edge of poverty, and its members' prospects of succeeding in the US economic system are not bright. Perhaps reflecting on this, many members do not view the current social-political system in a favourable light. Some of these sustainers may be attracted to the more spiritual and philosophical branches of CM, which they practice more out of interest than medical need. Further, minority or migrant groups may practice very unique or specific folk medicine treatments which are far outside the range of orthodox medicine.

The Outer-Directed Lifestyle (67% of the population)
This segment represents the mainstream of the population, with two out of three adults living in this type of lifestyle. The outstanding characteristics of this type is that other people are used as guides for both values and behaviours. Concern for the social implications and norms of behaviour is quite high for all three segments here, although they differ from each other in some other important ways.

"Belongers" constitute the largest VALS segment with almost 40 percent of the total population. They would rather "fit in" than "stand out". These are the stabilizers of society, a strong force for traditional values and behaviours. Family, church, and home are important to members of this segment. These individuals tend to be white, to be older than average, and to have somewhat lower levels of education and income than most other segments. Belongers are usually only prepared to believe in, or seek out, CM practice if it is endorsed by people and important figures in the community. That is, they adopt CM only if it becomes both fashionable and normative. Thus, in Britain they may well be enthusiastic about homoeopathy which has received Royal approval.

"Emulators" is a much smaller (8% of the population) and different group

Lifestyle, Beliefs and Value Systems 53

than Belongers. These people are young (average age 28) and are trying hard to "make it big" in the system. They are ambitious, competitive, and status conscious. Their lifestyles and value systems reflect (emulate) their aspirational reference group — the Achievers. Minorities are over-represented in this segment, the educational level is about average for all segments, and the income level is above that of Belongers but below that of Achievers. Unless those who they emulate expound CM approaches, this group is unlikely to do so. They are likely to be extremely fickle and capricious with regard to CM practices, picking them up, adopting them but equally discarding them at a rapid rate.

"Achievers" account for one-fifth of the population and include the leaders in business, the professionals, and government. These people are competent, successful, and hard-working. They tend to have materialistic values, are pleased with the economic system, and appear to be well satisfied with their place in society. Males are over-represented in this group and minorities are quite under-represented. Members are slightly older than average, have almost two years of college on average, and hold the highest family income level of any segment. By-and-large Achievers are not attracted to CM, though chronic medical problems or a discontent with orthodox medicine may induce them to investigate more well established branches of CM like homoeopathy or acupuncture.

The Inner-Directed Lifestyles (20% of the population)
The primary distinction between this lifestyle and the "outer-directed" majority lies in the fact that these people seem more concerned with resolving issues in their inner life than in dealing with the values of the external world. This does not mean that these people have rejected the lifestyles or value systems of the outer-directed. Instead, many of the people living in this lifestyle have been sufficiently successful that they have now chosen to pursue additional interests to that of economic success within the system.

"I-am-Me's" are individuals in a transition stage that lasts only for a few years and represents a mix of values from both inner- and outer-directed lifestyles. This is a very small segment (only 3 per cent of the population), but an interesting one through which many people pass. The average I-Am-Me is 20 years old, has slightly less than a high school degree (though many are still in college), and has a lower than average income (again as a result of the age of the group). People at this stage are fiercely individualistic, somewhat narcissistic, and somewhat exhibitionistic. Because they are very concerned with their inner identities and external potentials, they are often willing to try new activities, to take risks, and to act impulsively. It is quite likely that this group has a brief and passionate interest in more than one branch of CM though it might not last long. Further, it is more likely to be the fringe end of CM practice (e.g., crystals).

"Experientials" constitute another small segment (6 per cent of the population) which is also somewhat tied to a person's progress through the life cycle. Their average age is 26, they tend to be female and white, with higher than average educational levels and household incomes. This group is the most inner-directed of any of the segments and seeks personal involvement and experience with many aspects of life. Because CM offers the opportunity for experiential learning this group may well be very attracted to it. Indeed, the data do suggest that the average CM patient is white, middle class and middle aged. They have adopted a consumerist and often mildly feminist outlook.

"Societally conscious" individuals represent the farthest step along the VALS inner-directed path and constitute 11 per cent of the adult population. These people have extended their value system beyond themselves to include various concerns with improving (as they see it) society as a whole. This is undertaken not for personal gain in a materialistic sense, but because the person believes that "the world ought to be better than it is". Many of these individuals support causes such as conservation, and many engage in extensive volunteer work. These individuals tend to be late in their 30s on average and have high levels of education and income. Various branches of CM appear particularly attractive to this group because of the values they espouse. It is therefore highly likely that this group flirts with many branches of CM while devotedly following specific practices from one branch.

The "Integrated" Lifestyle (2 per cent of the population)
These are the rare "self-actualising individuals who represent the highest stage of the VALS system. Their values and lifestyles combine the power of the outer-directed achiever with the sensitivity of the inner-directed socially conscious individual. They are 40 years old on average, hold a college degree, and have a high income level. Because they account for only 2 per cent of the population, however, they are not a very significant segment for marketers aiming at the mass consumer market. However, they may well have fairly extensive experience with CM.

How does this system work? Consider Table 3 which is an application of VALS. It can be seen that the imported wine market is highly segmented. Survivors virtually never buy this product (they may instead drink domestic wines or not drink much wine at all) and the other segments at the top of the list are also buying imported wines at rates much below the national average. The segments towards the bottom of the list constitute "heavy users" of imported wines. Since Belongers are by far the largest segment, marketers might in this case, want to key in on this group to gain increased sales in the future.

The second column indicates the way in which competition occurs within a general use category. Notice that most segments buy cold cereals at about the national average, with Survivors and Emulators being lower, and the huge Belonger segment providing a massive sales base as they buy at higher than average rates.

The media columns show that it is possible to use VALS to segment markets according to their uses of media. This is important in the context of planning media campaigns and knowing where are the best media outlets to place commercial messages in order to reach target markets. The example in the table shows how highly segmented are the audiences for TV comedy shows. The same is also true of sports magazine readerships.

The final two columns indicate that VALS has been used to segment individuals on the basis of their activity and interest characteristics. The intriguing question remains whether one could accurately segment the CM market psychographically. Thus, one may have either CM vs orthodox, conventional medicine, or specific branches of CM like homoeopath, herbalism, acupuncture as columns. Although the analysis seems not to have been done, it is quite possible. Indeed, it may help to target the advertising and general proselytising of CM in general.

Table 3: VALS segments and consumer behaviour

| | Index of Purchase/Usage (national average rate = 1.0) ||||||
| | Products || Media || Activities ||
	Imported Wines	Cold Cereals	TV	General Sports Magazines	Fishing	Museums Galleries
Survivors (4%)	L(0.6)	L(0.8)	L(0.7)	L(0.0)	L(0.5)	L(0.4)
Sustainers (7%)	L(0.4)	-	H(2.0)	L(0.8)	H(2.0)	L(0.5)
Belongers (39%)	L(0.6)	H(1.3)	-	L(0.7)	H(1.3)	L(0.8)
Emulators (8%)	L(0.7)	L(0.7)	H(1.5)	H(1.2)	-	L(0.6)
Achievers (20%)	H(1.4)	-	L(0.7)	-	-	H(1.7)
I-Am-Me's (3%)	-	-	H(1.8)	H(2.0)	-	L(0.7)
Experientials (6%)	H(2.2)	-	H(1.4)	H(1.3)	-	H(1.3)
Societally Conscious (11%)	H(1.9)	-	L(0.7)	-	L(0.7)	H(1.9)

Source: T.C. Thomas & S. Crocker, *Values and Lifestyles – The New Psychographics* (Menlo Park, Calif: SRI International, 1981).

To be read:
"Survivors drink imported wine at a much lower (L) than average rate, only 0.6 of the national average. Sustainers, Belongers and Emulators also buy imported

wines at lower than average rates, while Achievers, Experientials, and Societally Conscious buy at higher (H) rates than the average. The I-Am-Me segment purchases imported wine at a rate close to the average (-)".

The VALS system has been updated and others introduced.

Social Value Groups

A British system has also been developed. Seven Social Value Groups have been produced from research marketed by UK market research agency, Taylor Nelson Ltd. The main purpose behind the Monitor system is to help companies respond to the general changes in social values that are taking place across any given period of time. Their repeated use over many years has enabled the system to be used as a source of value trends which can be applied to long-range planning and market formatting, as well as for brand positioning at any particular point in time. In all, seven types are described.

Self Explorers are youthful, independent, comfortably situated, often females. These are self-aware people who cannot tolerate restriction unless self-imposed. They are confident, tolerant, imaginative, and enjoy a secure, comfortable self-oriented lifestyle.

Social Register is an older group who resist change, seek to maintain the status quo. They have a high need for control over self, family, community, and society. Tend to seek to preserve traditional ethical and moral codes.

Experimentalists tend to be men in their late 20s, early 30s, independent and unconventional, and always looking for something new and different. They are energetic, confident, gregarious and intelligent, and work oriented.

Conspicuous Consumers are predominantly female office workers or housewives with a standard basic education. Essentially conformist with little need for personal satisfaction, their energy is directed toward romantic goals and material possessions. They generally lack self-confidence and mix with similarly oriented friends.

Belongers are mature, stable and settled; the most married group of all and likely to have a young family. They place great store by the home, family and country, establishment and fair play.

Survivors tend to be male, unskilled or skilled manual workers, dependent on the protection of authority while also sceptical of its intentions. These people identify with the country, family, trade unions or a political party; motivated by basic physical and emotional needs.

Aimless lack orientation within society, goalless, uninvolved and alienated.

Can be aggressive and resentful towards system's authority. Unhappy and unable to improve their position, may turn to fantasy and cheap 'kicks' for distraction.

Once again it is possible to speculate, or indeed, test hypotheses about relationships between these 7 groups and their attitudes to, knowledge of, or experience concerning CM and its many branches.

Medical Examples of Psychographic Segmentation

Psychographic or lifestyle segmentation has been applied to various medical products. Frequently, rather than use existing general classifications to segment the market for a particular product, psychographics has devised categories per product. Consider the following two points.

Prescription Drugs
Ziff (1971) surveyed 2000 housewives across the USA. They were given 214 attitude statements; their responses to these statements were factor analysed to produce a general classification of the group as a whole. Secondly, separate analyses were computed on selections of items dealing with specific food product categories: drugs, personal, and household items. She reports the classification for drug use only – among the product classifications. Four categories were derived:

Realists are not health fatalists, nor excessively concerned with protection or germs. They view remedies positively, want something that is convenient and works, and do not feel the need of a doctor-recommended medicine.

Authority Seekers are doctor and prescription oriented, are neither fatalists nor stoics concerning health, but they prefer the stamp of authority on what they do take.

Sceptics have a low health concern, are least likely to resort to medication, and are highly sceptical of cold remedies.

Hypochondriacs have a high health concern, regard themselves as prone to any bug going around, and tend to take medication at the first symptom. They do not look for strength in what they take, but need some mild authority reassurance.

In examining the relationships between product usage and segmentation solely derived from drug-related statements, Ziff found some interesting results. As expected Hypochondriacs were high in usage, the Sceptics were low, the Realists and Authority Seekers in between.

Stomach Remedy

Pernica (1971) reported on a market segmentation study of consumers of a stomach remedy. He developed a list of 80 items that included symptom frequency and benefits provided by different brands, attitudes toward treatment, and beliefs about ailments. Items tapping general personality traits were recast so as to be product specific. For instance, "I worry too much" was translated into "I seem to get stomach problems if I worry too much". The 80 product-specific items were reduced to 13 factors, and scores on the latter were obtained for each respondent. The resultant consumer segments, which are shown below, were described in terms of personality traits, lifestyle attributes, and demographic information about respondents. The outcome of this research was consistent with other studies. When segmentation is based upon the dimensions on which other brands differ, they were much more readily discriminable than when it was based on more general considerations.

The *Severe Sufferers* are the extreme group in the potency side of the market. They tend to be young, have children, and be well educated. They are irritable and anxious people and believe they suffer more severely than others. They take the ailments seriously, fuss about it, pamper themselves and keep trying new and different products.

The *Active Medicators* are on the same side of the motivational spectrum. They are typically modern suburbanites with average income and education. They are emotionally adjusted to the demands of their active lives. They use remedies to relieve every ache and pain.

The *Hypochondriacs* are on the opposite side of the motivational spectrum. They tend to be older, not as well educated, and women. They have conservative attitudes toward medication and a deep concern over health. They see possible dangers in frequent use of remedies, are concerned over side effects, and are afraid of remedies with new ingredients and extra potency. They are strongly oriented toward medical authority, seeking guidance in treatment.

The *Practicalists* are in the extreme position on this side of the motivational spectrum. They tend to be older, well educated, emotionally the most stable, and least concerned over their ailment or the dangers of remedies. They accept the ailment and its discomforts as a part of life, without fuss and pampering. They use a remedy as a last resort.

The Advantages and Disadvantages of Psychographic Analysis

How sensitive, accurate and reliable is a psychographic analysis of products or user groups? Is it really more useful for a simple public relations exercise? Whilst it may appeal to those in marketing has it anything to offer researchers in alternative medicine? In short are psychographic studies useful? There is strong disagreement on this point. Some users have been pleased with the studies they have conducted and believe that psychographics represents a major breakthrough in consumer research. Others have been disappointed with their experiences with psychographics and believe it to be a waste of time and money. Some believe that product-specific psychographic studies are extremely valuable, but that general lifestyle studies are useless; while others believe the opposite.

Critics of psychographics (Gunter & Furnham 1992) generally base their criticisms on the following points:

1. The groups of consumers, users or "believers" created by psychographic analysis overlap so much that they do not differentiate among consumer types.
2. The length of many, if not most, psychographic questionnaires precludes obtaining a probability sample; thus the findings are non-representative and cannot be projected onto wider population groups.
3. Psychographic studies reveal nothing that shrewd marketing practitioners, creative advertising, or astute researcher writers do not already know or could not figure out if they just bothered to think about it.
4. Psychographics is just another gimmick that has a certain naive appeal but no real substance.

Devout users of psychographics generally support its value with the following arguments:

1. Granted that life-cycle, lifestyle and product-loyal groups overlap substantially, the marginal differences that exist can still be useful because differences of only a couple of percentage points are routinely used in making marketing decisions.
2. Psychographic studies provide insights into the behaviour of consumers that cannot be obtained in any other way, and these studies often inspire concepts and ideas that substantially strengthen the marketing effort.

3. Psychographics is a powerful selling tool in helping advertising agencies obtain clients, marketing personnel sell their recommendations to corporate management and researchers understand the differences between groups.

Comprehensive reviews of psychographics and market segmentation research, such as *Lifestyle and Psychographics* edited by Wells (1974), and the special section on market segmentation research of the *Journal of Marketing Research* edited by Wind (1978), have levelled the following conceptual and operational criticisms at psychographic research:

1. The validity of market segmentation solutions cannot be ascertained because of the limited theory.
2. Segmentation descriptors which are chosen because they richly describe should not necessarily be expected to predict well.
3. Lifestyle and psychographic dimensions may have added to the predictive ability of demographics, but their relationships with consumer behaviour have been far from impressive.
4. By attempting to analyse 'everything with everything', psychographic market segmentation practice is merely an exploratory first stage of the research process.
5. Because of limited theoretical development, psychographics research ignores the hierarchy of effects of learning behaviour consumers go through in making decisions.
6. Since adequate psychographic theory has not been developed, the selection of segmentation descriptors and scales is too often a 'fishing expedition'.

In its defence, psychographics have been used frequently because of the rich descriptive detail they have provided to developing marketing strategies and research hypotheses. Numerous testimonials exist attesting to how the descriptive detail of psychographic research enhanced development of corporate marketing strategy.

Unlike demographics, many social and psychological factors are difficult to measure, being somewhat objective, usually based on the self-reports of consumers and sometimes hidden from view (to avoid embarrassment, protect privacy, convey an image and other reasons). In addition, there are still ongoing disputes over terminology, misuse of data and reliability.

One of the pioneers of this area of research, William D. Wells, highlighted the problems and limitations of this approach to market segmentation:

"From the speed with which psychographics have diffused through the marketing community, it seems obvious that they are perceived as meeting a keenly felt need. The problem now is not so much one of pioneering as it is one of sorting out the techniques that work best. As that process proceeds, it seems extremely likely that psychographic methods will gradually become more familiar and less controversial, and eventually will merge into the mainstream of marketing research" (Wells 1975: 209).

What is the difference between the way applied marketers and academics use psychographic and lifestyle analyses? Do medical and social scientists use the term differently in research? How is lifestyle analysis used in complementary medicine research?

Probably the most striking difference between applied and academic researchers is the terms they use. The latter often use technical terms based on specific theories like locus of control or attribution style. Related to this is the fact that whereas applied marketeers tend to aim to describe people in terms of *types*, social science and medical practitioners, particularly the former, use *trait dimensions*. Social scientists talk in terms of types like introvert and extravert but actually measure along dimensions. However, there is a tradition in medicine, particularly psychiatry, that has preferred the "case-ness" of types.

Both applied and academic researchers like to use established dimensions or category systems (like VALS) but the former are less rigid in the application of one system for all issues. However, academic researchers do yearn for universality and thus would not approve of the segmentation or descriptions of groups of people or patients in terms of one product or service that they favoured. That is, academic researchers would attempt to examine which features of lifestyles (values, beliefs, behaviours) were associated with choice and use of which specific (from the full range) of alternative therapies. The idea is to get, and understand, the best predictors of a choice of medical practitioners, not to describe how many of type A, B, or C usually go to them.

Social scientists, in attempting to investigate the world of complementary medicine, have already a rich bank of concepts and research. Traditionally, what they would do is review the literature; select a number of promising variables thought to relate to the behaviour or beliefs examined; derive quite specific and testable hypotheses and then do an analysis. Further, their techniques like multiple regression would probably be different than applied researchers because of the sort of questions that they would ask.

Can lifestyle or psychographic analysis help in the understanding of people's attitudes toward, knowledge about, belief in, and ultimately experience of CM?

The answer is probably yes. Products, services, and philosophies can all be subject to the basic approach of lifestyle analysis. However, whether one should use a general inventory like VALS, or devise a product/service-specific measure is uncertain.

What the subject does offer, however, is a way of looking at CM-related behaviours within the whole context of the individual. Because lifestyle analysis looks at *categories* of lifestyle, it allows certain beliefs and behaviours to be embedded in a wider context which may help understand the aetiology and maintenance of the behaviour and belief in the first place.

Personal Values and Complementary Medicine

For over 40 years psychologists have attempted to read people's value systems. For Rokeach (1973) as for Feather (1990) a value is an enduring belief that a specific instrumental mode of conduct or terminal end state of existence is preferable.

> "Once a value is internalized it becomes, consciously or unconsciously, a standard or criterion for guiding action, for developing and maintaining attitudes toward relevant objects and situations, for justifying one's own and other's actions and attitudes, for morally judging self and others, and for comparing self with others" (Feather 1975: 16).

Values then are motives that involve normative considerations of 'oughtness' and desirability. They also serve as standards that guide behaviour and are linked to affect particularly when values are achieved or frustrated. Various societal institutions—the church, educational institutions—as well as the family and the media, shape (enhance, maintain, transmit) these values from one generation to the next. Thus, for researchers a person's value system must to a large extent reflect past socialization. Furthermore, the extent and direction of a change of values must reflect different fairly profound socialization experiences.

As well as educational differences, Feather (1975) has demonstrated that values are coherently and systematically related to age, sex, income, religious and socio-political beliefs and cultural differences. Although a lot of this work is descriptive and rarely specifically hypothesis-testing, most of the results are perfectly explicable and few counter-intuitive. As Feather (1990) noted, it is not possible to infer that values determine vocational or disciplinary choice.

"Causal sequences are difficult to specify ... Once a student has made his choice he probably begins to internalize some of the values, attitudes and behavioural patterns that he believes are characteristic of the School he joins ... Thus although he may have made his choice on the basis of other considerations, his ranking of the values may be according to his concept of how a typical Humanities, Social Science or Science student would rank them; that is, his value rankings may have resulted from his decision and his concept of a stereotype rather than the reverse" (Feather 1990: 138).

In a relevant study, Furnham (1988) looked at the terminal and instrumental values of three groups of first-year students: nursing, medical and psychology. There were a number of differences in the terminal values.

Table 4: Average values for the three groups for the terminal values and analysis of various differences

Terminal values	Group means			
	Medical students, $N = 74$	Nursing students, $N = 67$	Psychology students, $N = 52$	ANOVA
A COMFORTABLE LIFE (a prosperous life)	11.41(14)	12.53(16)	12.07(15)	1.05
AN EXCITING LIFE (a stimulating, active life)	6.29 (3)	8.43(6)	7.23(5)	3.64*
A SENSE OF ACCOMPLISHMENT (lasting contribution)	8.24 (8)	7.68(5)	10.36(13)	5.31**
A WORLD AT PEACE (free of war and conflict)	10.60 (12)	9.16(9)	8.42(7)	3.46*
A WORLD OF BEAUTY (beauty of nature and the arts)	13.02 (16)	11.56(13)	12.46(16)	2.48
EQUALITY (brotherhood, equal opportunity for all)	11.18 (13)	11.77(14)	9.75(11)	2.59
FAMILY SECURITY (taking care of loved ones)	9.45 (10)	6.91(3)	9.35(9)	3.89*
FREEDOM (independence and free choice)	6.95 (4)	7.01(4)	6.48(4)	0.21
HAPPINESS (contentedness)	4.77 (1)	3.58 (1)	5.57 (1)	3.68*
INNER HARMONY (free from inner conflict)	8.05 (6)	8.67 (7)	7.57 (6)	0.77
MATURE LOVE (sexual and spiritual intimacy)	7.20 (5)	9.17 (10)	6.28 (3)	7.11***
NATIONAL SECURITY (protection from attack)	15.01 (18)	14.82 (18)	15.40 (18)	0.65
PLEASURE (an enjoyable, leasurely life)	10.59 (11)	10.52 (12)	10.19 (12)	0.16
SALVATION (saved, eternal life)	14.29 (17)	11.83 (15)	14.69 (17)	4.08**
SELF-RESPECT (self-esteem)	8.12 (7)	9.14 (8)	8.65 (8)	4.08**
SOCIAL RECOGNITION (respect, admiration)	11.93 (15)	12.76 (17)	11.44 (14)	1.94
TRUE FRIENDSHIP (close companionship)	5.10 (2)	5.20 (2)	5.96 (2)	1.46
WISDOM (a mature understanding of life)	8.98 (9)	9.85 (11)	9.36 (10)	0.76

***$p < 0.001$; **$p < 0.01$; *$p < 0.05$. – Numbers in parentheses are rank orders.

Seven of the 18 values yielded significant differences. Medical students valued an *exciting life* higher than psychology students who in turn valued it higher than nursing students. Nursing students valued a *sense of accomplishment* more than medical students who in turn valued it significantly higher than psychology students. Both psychology and nursing students rate a *world at peace* higher than medical students. Nursing students rated *family security* higher than the two other groups who did not significantly differ from each other. Nursing students rated *happiness* higher than medical students who in turn rated it higher than psychology students. The biggest differences between the three groups occurred on the terminal value *mature love* which was rated highest by psychology students, and less by nursing students. Finally, the nursing students rated *salvation* higher than either of the other two groups.

Table 5: Average values for the three groups for the instrumental values and analysis of various differences

Terminal values	Group means			
	Medical students, N = 74	Nursing students, N = 67	Psychology students, N = 52	ANOVA
AMBITIOUS (hard-working, aspiring)	10.52(13)	10.77(13)	10.71(13)	0.04
BROADMINDED (open-minded)	7.36(4)	8.61(7)	6.73(3)	2.58
CAPABLE	8.75(7)	10.41(11)	8.62(9)	3.87*
CHEERFUL (light-hearted, joyful)	7.18(3)	5.16(3)	7.84(6)	6.70***
CLEAN (neat, tidy)	14.97(18)	12.88(16)	14.78(17)	5.82**
COURAGEOUS (standing up for your beliefs)	9.46(10)	10.13(10)	9.67(11)	0.38
FORGIVING (willing to pardon others)	8.79(8)	7.74(6)	8.76(10)	1.13
HELPFUL (working for the welfare of others)	8.36(6)	6.95(4)	8.61(8)	2.61
HONEST (sincere, truthful)	5.28(1)	4.91(2)	5.36(2)	0.23
IMAGINATIVE (daring, creative)	11.59(15)	13.14(17)	10.01(12)	3.76*
INDEPENDENT (self-reliant, self-sufficient)	8.85(9)	10.07(9)	8.09(7)	2.27
INTELLECTUAL (intelligent, reflective)	10.10(11)	11.47(14)	7.82(5)	8.43***
LOGICAL (consistent, rational)	11.18(14)	13.35(18)	12.90(16)	5.88**
LOVING (affectionate, tender)	5.55(2)	4.68(1)	4.11(1)	2.06
OBEDIENT (dutiful, respectful)	14.31(17)	12.86(15)	15.63(18)	7.87***
POLITE (courteous, well-mannered)	14.31(16)	10.50(12)	12.75(15)	3.90*
RESPONSIBLE (dependable, reliable)	7.70(5)	7.48(5)	7.35(4)	0.13
SELF-CONTROLLED (restrained, self-disciplined)	10.12(12)	9.29(8)	12.30(14)	3.26*

***$p<0.001$; **$p<0.01$; *$p<0.05$.

Half of the 18 instrumental values showed significant differences between the three groups. Both psychology and medical students rated *capable* higher, but *cheerful* and *clean* less highly than nursing students. Psychology students rated *imaginative* and *intellectual* higher than nursing students. Medical students rated *logical* higher than either nursing or psychology students. Nursing students rated *obedient* higher than medical students who in turn rated it higher than psychology students. Finally, nursing students rated *polite* and *self-controlled* significantly higher than medical students who in turn rated them higher than psychology students.

Furnham (1988) was aware that the problem with the study of value or personality differences between different occupations is that one cannot be sure whether the differences occurred before choosing a job (predispositional) or while being trained (socialization). In this study, for all practical purposes, it is possible to eliminate the socialization factor as the students had only just begun their courses. But he notes:

> "Finally the consequences of these value differences may be questioned both while undergoing their formal training, but also afterwards when and if they were working as professionals. Firstly it is not certain whether the socialization experience of training would reinforce or change the values held by all the students at the beginning of their training. Only longitudinal research could determine this. If however one can assume that these value differences are maintained the question remains as to whether these value differences have a beneficial or deleterious effect on communications, trust, etc., between these three groups. It is quite likely that people with radically different value systems would dislike, distrust and devalue each other. There is ample evidence to show how values relate to social action and interaction. Hence it may be expected that part of the difficulty experienced by medical and paramedical professionals working together in case teams is a result of their different value priorities, that led them in the first place to choose one vocation over another. There is, after all, no mystery about where the value constellations of the various groups originate. All three groups (doctors, psychologists, nurses) have different power bases in systems of medical care, enjoy different monetary rewards and, in spite of recent attempts at egalitarian blurring, still bear vastly different kinds of responsibility. No group is more acutely aware of those hierarchies than apprentices. Nor are nascent professionals aware of the differences in their historical legacies however uninformed about the facts of these roots they may be. In short, the occupational fields which are the object of this research have a

history which must, in part, be a determinant of the values they espouse" (Furnham 1988: 619).

This study merely illustrates some of the more important issues relevant to the relationship between values and choice of CM. First, it is quite probable that people who choose and use CM practitioners exclusively or primarily have different values than those who use orthodox practitioners. Equally, it is possible that the practitioners of the two different branches of medicine hold different values. Thus, one could speculate that orthodox patients and practitioners value logic, obedience, self-control, accomplishment and freedom above CM patients and practitioners, who in turn value imagination, beauty, security, and salvation higher.

However, even if one was to find these predicted statistically significant differences, it remains unclear as to whether value differences led to patients/practitioners choosing the particular branch of CM, or whether the experience of that type of medicine led to the value differences. Indeed, what is more probable is that the effect is bi-directional — there are both predispositional and socialization effects.

Furnham and Vincent (1995) in fact compared the values of patients of an orthodox medical GP and a complementary homoeopathic practitioner. Only 7 (of 27) terminal values clearly discriminated between the groups. Homoeopathic patients seem to value *dignity*, *salvation* and *national greatness* above the GP patients, who seem to value *mature love, a good life for others, personal support* and *wisdom* more. Homoeopathic patients appear to endorse ideological values more, while GP patients valued personal issues. Only five instrumental values discriminated between the two groups: homoeopathic patients valued *resourceful, tactful, ambitious* and *giving others a fair go* more than GP patients, who in turn valued *refined*.

In fact, no differences emerged in those areas that might be thought to be associated with the philosophy of complementary medicine. Homoeopathy involves a detailed history in which great attention is paid to emotional factors; its underlying theory emphasizes emotional and physical balance and harmony, yet values such as *inner harmony* and *self-knowledge* did not distinguish the two groups.

These preliminary results suggest that there are few basic value differences between patients attending complementary and orthodox practitioners, although there could well be value differences between orthodox and complementary practitioners themselves. It may well be that people are misinterpreting 'New Age' beliefs, which are in accordance with many modern orthodox beliefs. Thus, as Coward (1989) points out, New Age therapies' view of the person interprets individuals as essentially capable of good health *and* mental adjustment if only they are prepared to take responsibility for their own health. As Sharma (1992) notes, because these New Age ideas are not as radical as many assume, patients may start out using non-orthodox treatments, holding health beliefs and values which are no different from users, but their very exposure to the ideas of the therapist may effect such a change over time.

Assuming that this effect can be replicated, it seems that reviewers who have suggested that patients of complementary practitioners are distinguished by an adherence to a New Age philosophy or have distinct world views are probably wrong. Although it is possible that some patients are attracted to a particular branch of CM purely, or even predominately, on the basis of its philosophy or espoused value system, other factors clearly play a more important role. Many prospective patients are unaware of the philosophy and value underpinning their chosen branch of alternative medicine. Rather, their choices are pragmatic.

Conclusion

This paper focuses on one "hypothesis" for researchers interested in CM. Many have agreed that the beliefs, values or lifestyle of people lead them to be attracted to CM (and indeed, orthodox medical treatment). That is, patients seek an ideological "fit" between their own system and that espoused by the particular CM speciality. This seems an altogether quite reasonable assumption. However, the literature shows that there are numerous difficult problems.

First, not only is the concept of lifestyle difficult to operationalize and measure, it is simply tautological to imply that lifestyle somehow accounts for the choice of CM. The marketing literature on psychographics is interesting and shows how patient groups may be described in terms of their choice of particular medicines or therapies. However interesting and descriptive psychographics is, it is psychometrically weak, seems very confined to particular products or population groups and more importantly appears not to explain the process or mechanism whereby people seek out a particular CM practice.

Secondly, the literature on value systems seems to suggest that whilst their values may determine why practitioners become particular CM practitioners, value differences are not closely related to patients' beliefs. There remains more work to be done in the areas certainly, but it is possible that except on the most general level, patients are not well informed about the numerous and subtle values espoused by different areas of CM.

The current research in this area appears to indicate that CM patients are not anti-scientific, ideologically driven individuals but pragmatic shoppers for health. They appear not to be "brand loyal" to medicine of any kind. Few patients are exclusive users of one branch of complementary medicine. Most people have an understanding that certain types of complementary medicine are ideally suited to specific complaints. Equally, they believe orthodox medicine to be by far the most efficient for problems associated with broken bones, bleeding etc. The more health options available, the more people shop for health, trying out various solutions or cures to different conditions. There is more evidence that this is the case. This seems particularly true of very health-conscious people.

But by far the most important explanation for the choice of CM is dissatisfaction with orthodox medicine, which has either failed them in particular or not adapted to the differing needs of the new consumerist patient.

There is considerably more evidence to support this type of explanation, which holds that patients of alternative practitioners have had bad experiences with orthodox doctors. These experiences come in a number of forms: first that the doctor does not seem to take the time or care to "fully understand" the patient. That is, that patients feel they are being processed too quickly by the orthodox medical system. They are rarely examined (touched) and their feelings rarely discussed. They feel cheated; possibly their expectations from a consultation are inappropriate and unreasonable; also they may be presenting obviously psychosomatic or trivial complaints that busy orthodox doctors cannot deal with. Another reason for dissatisfaction lies in the patient's perception that the doctor and his/her cure/therapy simply does not work. That is, chronic conditions, most frequently back pains, get no better and the orthodox practitioner for all his/her training and the advancement of modern medicine is unable to deal with the problem. Despite the development of high-tech medicine, many patients find it is clearly unable to deal with their simple but chronic illnesses.

Thirdly, there are patients who fear orthodox medical practitioners. They fear their power and their methods, which some see as too technological and insufficiently sensitive to individual differences. Surgeons frequently epitomise the all-powerful, even brutal, side of medicine. Studies on the health locus of control show that orthodox medical patients have more faith in their practitioner, but also take less responsibility for their own health. It really revolves around the issues of trust and the extent to which patients believe their practitioners can and do help them.

In many Western countries the consumer, ecological and feminist movements have all socialized people into dealing rather differently with professionals, be they accountants, lawyers or doctors. They want a different kind of relationship, but modern medicine appears to have, in part, ignored that message. Through ignorance, arrogance, or simply increased pressure on their services, many orthodox practitioners have changed their attitudes and behaviours little with respect to the patient. Hence, they have alienated a generation of those wanting more from their medical practitioner. Thus, they are not drawn so much by the claims of CM practitioners, but the way in which they treat their patients. It is the quality of the relationship rather than ideology or lifestyle that is apparently the best predictor of why patients choose and stay with medical practitioners of all persuasions.

References

Backett, K. & Davison, C.
1995 "Life course and lifestyle", in: *Social Science and Medicine*, 40: 629-638.

Blackwell, R. & Talarzyk, D.
1977 "Lifestyle retailing: competition strategies for the 1980s", in: *Journal of Retailing*, 59: 7-27.

Cathelat, B.
1993 *Socio-Styles*, Kogan Page: London.

Cosmas, S.
1982 "Life style and consumption patterns", in: *Journal of Consumer Research*, 8: 453-455.

Coward, R.
1989 *The Whole Truth: The myth of alternative health*, Routledge: London.

Davison, C., Frankel, S. & Smith, C.
1992 "The limits of lifestyle", in: *Social Science and Medicine*, 34: 675-685.

Demby, E.
1974 "Psychographics and from whence it came", in: W. Wells (ed.): *Life Style and Psychographics*, AMA: Chicago.

Feather, N.
1975 *Values and Education in Society*, Free Press: New York.
1990 *Expectations and Actions: Expectancy-Value Models in Psychology*, Lawrence Erlbaum: New York.

Furnham, A.
1988 "Values and vocational choice", in: *Social Science and Medicine*, 26: 613-617.

Furnham, A. & Vincent, C.
1995 "Value differences in orthodox and complementary medicine patients", in: *Complementary Therapies in Medicine*, 3: 65-69.

Gunter, B. & Furnham, A.
1992 *Consumer Profiles: An introduction to psychographics*, Routledge: London.

Mitchell, A.
1983 *The Nine American Life Styles*, Warner: New York.

Pernica, J.
1971 "Psychographics: What can go wrong", in: R. Carhan (ed.): *Combined Proceedings of the American Marketing Association*, pp. 45-50.

Plummer, J.
1974 "The concept and application of life style segmentation", in: *Journal of Marketing*, 38: 33-37.

Reynolds, F. & Darden, W.
1974 "An analysis of selected factors associated with the adoption of new products", in: *Mississippi Valley Journal of Business and Economics*, 8: 31-42.

Riesman, D., Glazer, N. & Denney, R.
1950 *The Lonely Crowd*, Yale University Press: New Haven, CT.

Rokeach, M.
1973 *The Nature of Human Values*, Free Press: New York.

Sharma, U.
1992 *Complementary Medicine Today: Practitioners and Patients*, Routledge: London.

Wells, W.
1974 *Life Style and Psychographics*, AMA: Chicago.
1975 "Psychographics: A critical view", in: *Journal of Marketing Research*, 12: 209-229.

Wind Y.
1978 "Issues and advances in segmentation research", in: *Journal of Marketing Research*, 15, 317-337.

Ziff, R.
1971 "Psychographics for market segmentation", in: *Journal of Advertising Researching*, 11: 3-10.

Coping with Emotions and Stress of Life

by Nelly Tsouyopoulos

The vision of the doctor with the competence to instruct people in the lessons of living is based on the assumption of the inseparable connection between moral and medical duties. Physiology as the science of human nature appears thus to be the foundation of ethics and of life code. The equation of health with virtue was not invented by contemporary health education, which only reinforces a very deep-seated concept (Blaxter 1995: 243). Today, we are rather critical about the expansion of medicine to needs that go beyond the training and ability of most physicians. Nevertheless, we believe there is considerable value in health promotion and in disease prevention, but we see the value of the prevention not only in the technology which tries to find the beginning of a disease as early as possible, but also in making people more involved in self-care. If we want to avoid the total medicalization of life and the physician becoming the central healer of society, we have to take the challenge of our time in reforming our responsibility for self-care. On the other hand, we do not agree with those health promoters who suggest that the well-being and health of individuals is a product of their lifestyles. Bodily function is central for health and it is mainly a matter of medicine. The ideology which places the responsibility for health squarely upon the individual himself is counter-productive. The suggestion that diseases are due to the lifestyles of the sufferers brings forth the issue of culpability (Davison and Darey Smith 1995: 92). Health promotion and self-care have to be compatible with the main principles of physiology.

Self-Care and The Mind-Body Problem

The most important question in physiology from the point of view of self-care is the question of overcoming the division between mind and body, because self-care implies a holistic concept of the person. Several scientific investigations of modern physiology can give an answer to this fundamental question: Scientific medicine does not ignore the old principle of hippocratic medicine, the healing force of nature, the *vis medicatrix naturae*, according to which processes of restoration of health after disease and of repair after injury go on independently of any medical treatment. According to this idea, the body acts as a subject, intentional and with regard to the whole organism; the ability of repairing the injuries, the process of restoration of health cannot be understood without a plan. The idea that disease is cured by a *vis medicatrix naturae* implies the existence of agencies that are ready to operate correctively when the normal state of the organism is deranged. We, thus, refer to self-regulatory or self-controlling or self-rectifying processes.

Now, what do we mean by the word "self" in these expressions? Indeed, if we want to differentiate between several living processes, this "self" is a very important criterion. For every one of these activities regarded as self-regulation has a special distance from the "self" regarded as the watcher of this activity. In the case of the person trying to control his thoughts there is no distance at all. The watcher of this activity identifies himself with the "self" that controls this process of thinking. Other self-controlled activities of the organism, again, such as the respiratory process only partly allow the above identification. The watcher of the activity may sometimes be the subject, indicated by the process of self-regulation, for example, by initiating deeper and deeper breathing; but the whole economy of the process seems to be maintained by agencies to which the watcher has a clear distance. The watcher cannot identify himself here with the "self" of self-regulation, which remains active even if the watcher is excluded, as happens during sleeping. There are also other processes that are self-controlled activities, but they are not even perceived by the watcher, so that the subject of the activity seems to be quite different from the self, acting as watcher. If the skin, for example, is broken, connective tissue cells develop as supporting structures, thus making the region as durable as before. The self can watch this wonderful activity of self-repairing, or if it is not possible, it can be informed about it through lectures or reading books; in any case, it has no direct knowledge of it and no idea about the agencies engaged in this process. On the other hand, the watcher knows that all these activities are his own activities and that he cannot have a real knowledge of himself without having understood the various activities and processes as a whole. Self-knowledge is indeed the most difficult kind of knowledge, as all philosophers have taught. The fact that the watcher is only in part the agent of the activities that constitute his own life led to the crucial division between voluntary and involuntary processes of the living beings (Tsouyopoulos 1988). The physiologist, W. Cannon, who studied experimentally the rectifying tendency of organisms, called this ability to recover and reestablish a constant situation after disturbance, the "wisdom of the body". Cannon nevertheless thought that this ability has nothing to do with our consciousness or will, but a special part of the autonomic nervous system, the sympathicoadrenal division, is charged with the performance of these services, quite outside conscious direction (Cannon 1947: 297). The suggested autonomy of the system that is responsible for our stability has since become a dogma of medical anthropology and put a barrier between the voluntary and involuntary processes, and between the body and self-knowledge. For medicine, Cannon's theory means an essential change from the old crude reductive mechanism to a neo-mechanism, which allows a more exact reduction of the phenomena to quantitative values. Because of the wisdom of the body, modern medicine can obtain quantitative mean values regarding temperature, blood pressure, salt content in blood, etc. These are considered to give the normal situation of the organism, while any deviation from these indicates abnormality.

The concepts of normal and normality, however, are axiological and it is therefore doubtful whether the real meaning is preserved if we identify abnormal with quantitative deviation. The definition and classification of disease is to some extent socially constructed and normality itself is a relative and judgmental concept. It is obvious that the relevance of a pathological situation does not lie in the deviation of a statistical mean value, but in the fact that the situation is disadvantageous for the sick person and therefore has to be changed.

According to Georges Canguilhem, life, as such, is intentional and therefore a normative activity. Canguilhem's concept of "normativity" suggesting intentionality and purposiveness of life, can be considered to be a regulative idea similar to Cannon's "wisdom of the body". But Cannon's regulative principle is conceived as a rectifying mechanism of the body that works according to the law of flowing equilibria. According to Canguilhem, life has not only the rectifying tendency, the ability to recover and reestablish a constant situation after disturbance, but it can elaborate new norms. And that is why life can be called normative (Canguilhelm 1972: 77). Meanwhile observations, experiments and especially representatives of oriental cultures have shown that there is no obstacle, nothing to prevent communication between voluntary and involuntary processes (Hirai 1978).

The Concept of Stress

The concept of stress which Selye had developed in his early studies in the 1950s, is very similar to Canguilhem's concept of normativity. His investigations of the general adaptation syndrome supports the hypothesis that the organism responds to the environmental challenge as a whole; and that this response is not a mere reaction to the stressor, but an interpretation of it. What disturbs the organism and makes it sick is not the stressor as such, but the way the living being understands it. Consequently, important for health and disease is not the objective cause, but our own emotions and thoughts about some objective situation. The body can meet various aggressions with the same defensive reaction. This has psychosomatic implications. Bodily changes during stress act upon psychical and mental situations and vice versa (Selye 1975: 367). Whatever we do in coping with our world and problems, our whole activity is involved. Therefore, our health and disease can only be understood as a part of our whole self. Stress anyhow is not identical with stressors; neither physical nor psychosocial events can be causes of stress. If, for example, driving is thought to be a stressor, it is obvious that the objective fact "driving" cannot be the cause of any disturbance in the organism; for there are millions of people who drive without any stress. Those again, who, without any special reason, are stressed in traffic, can cope with other complex and dangerous activities without stress. Contrary situations can stress people: some are stressed in crowded places, while others are stressed when they are left alone with themselves. Therefore, it is not meaningful to say that life-events such as divorce or widowhood or unemployment are particular forms of stress and as such causes of increased risk of morbidity or mortality. For in this way we make out of stress theory a model of disease similar to that of infectious diseases; instead of microbes and viruses we consider migration or job change as causes of certain diseases.

The belief that there is a close relationship between stress and health is a long tradition in our society. Most people are well aware of the evidence that the reaction to prolonged stress can include physiological effects, specific or more generally, upon the immune system. But the concept of stress as a cause of ill health in one's life makes people seek an excuse for themselves in their feeling under stress, rather than try to cope with it. In all stress-situations there are emotions involved. But we know that emotions do not emerge without some thoughts and evaluations of our situation. Each time we lose our balance or we cannot solve our problems, we realize that our perceptions are coloured with emotions. We are also acquainted with the physical sensation in the abdomen that slowly spreads over the chest, or the tight feeling in the throat when we are overcome by emotion. On the other hand, we know that if we try to remain calm and be mindful of the present moment, we can dominate our emotions. So the stress theory, which was developed at the same time as the investigations about voluntary control, supports the expectations of a better understanding of the relationship between the will, the emotions and the involuntary activities of the body.

In summary, modern physiology suggests that our organism exists on the ground of self-regulating stability and of an intrinsic healing power, and that not only our thoughts and emotions but also our judgements and evaluation of our situation can cause changes in all processes and regulatory mechanisms of our organic system. Thus, the scientific knowledge of modern medicine is compatible with the idea of self-care, which is grounded on the possibility that conscious efforts can influence the activity of organic processes and promote health and well-being of our self.

Emotions and Emotional Stress

Some philosophers have seen in emotions and affections a disturbance of the soul, something analogous to the sickness of the body. For the stoics the affected soul loses its balance and becomes sick (Reesor 1989: 143). Descartes, who in modern philosophy studied the emotions very intensively, considers them to be the bridge between mind and body. The will has some power over them but it is not always capable of influencing emotional situations because of the simultaneous irritation in blood and brain activity (Descartes 1984: 205, article 136). Although Descartes' philosophy gave the foundation of dualism to medical thought, his study of affections and emotions gave rise to psychosomatic and holistic tendencies in medical treatment. Descartes' final judgement about emotions is that everything beautiful and sweet but also everything bitter in life is related to the emotions; people who are capable of deep feelings and emotional attachment can attain the richest experience in life (Descartes 1984: 325, article 212).

Nevertheless, our feelings are not always positive, and it is not easy to influence them. Emotional cycles and habit patterns are difficult to break. People develop a sense of hopelessness, a feeling that there is no alternative, no way out. Eventually, such an attitude causes loss of vitality or total indifference. Therefore, it is important to recognize the power of our emotions – and to take responsibility for them. There are times when the stress from our worries, fears and memories, constricts our energy to the point where we harm our own bodies or minds. Often, a latent disease tendency is transformed into a manifest malady by too much stress and strain. Emotional stress is the most harmful kind of stress. It has mostly to do with frustration and this is perhaps the point at which we can help ourselves. We cannot avoid stress because it is part of our lives; we cannot avoid every emotional situation but we can exercise to transform emotional stress which makes our lives unhealthy and unhappy. Emotions are the best way to know ourselves, to know our bodies, so coping with our emotions is the way of eliminating stress and of supporting our health.

Scientific medical ideas are compatible, as we saw, with holistic principles of self-care, but traditional patterns and prejudices make people neglect self-knowledge. Self-help is a way open to everyone, but self-education is not easy to attain; there are many and difficult obstacles to overcome. For example:

a) We have to reattain the ability to experience. This is difficult because our education in abstract thinking is one-sided. Methods of uniformity are much stronger than those of self-education. Conformism deprives us of our creativity and spontaneity; so we lose the interest and the ability to react to the diverse and complicated stimuli of our environment and of our intrinsic life. Our lifestyle is not always the result of our free choice. Even behaviour presumed to be voluntary, which represents deliberate choices about particular ways of living, may be imposed by family, economic or social situations. We live in a world that moves very fast and that pressures us to keep up. Very often, we do not want to live this way but we have been caught up by the demands society places on our lives. Sometimes we do not have the time to touch real life, so we lose the capacity of experience. So we know our emotions only by their results (crying, tears, depression). Our self-observation is but a process of introspective analysis and interpretation. We have to learn to recognize the circumstances that arouse emotions, to mobilize our resources; instead of causal analysis we must be able to have the experience of the emotional situation, of how emotion arises and manifests itself in body and mind.

b) Another difficulty we have to overcome is our resistance to change. Most of our patterns are supporting our identity as something unchangeable. We consider everything which happens to us, to our bodies and minds as reversible (Selye 1975: 429). We are thinking about irreversibility as identical with degeneration. But processes connected with time are irreversible, reality is irreversible. Knowing ourselves nevertheless implies the ability to change the established patterns and habits of body, feeling, mind. In short, the difficulty of learning lies less in the nature of the new, than in the resistance to the change of the established; any change of ourselves can be painful, because it is connected with the fear of losing identity. In order to change the mode of our action we have to change the image of ourselves.

The fear of losing our identity which we imagine to be something stable and unchangeable, is the most usual and difficult obstacle for coping with our emotional stress. Potential stressors are numerous: external, like offenses, challenges, rejection, indifference towards our person; but also internal, like unpleasant thoughts or memories. All these are met with emotional defensive responses. We hold on to emotional responses, even the negatives ones, because they form a major part of our identity. Letting go of them can be very frightening and confusing for without these familiar feelings we may no longer be sure who we are. Frustration stems from the need to act the role of who we are not. We must learn not to avoid or to push out emotions with unpleasant quality, but remain centered in immediate experience and try to change our perspective. We must also learn to adjust proportion between active defensive attitudes and measures of changing ourselves, in the best interest of maintaining our balance, which is a basic condition of our health. The philosophy of self-care is not different from the philosophy of self-knowledge. In both cases the ability to change in active and creative ways is essential.

We live today longer than at any other time before, but longer life alone is no value as such, for today's prevailing image of the aged is one of dependency. The increasing numbers of people who live into old age are defined as a social problem rather than as an achievement of the late 20th century (Hepwarth 1995: 182). Even if we accept the reality that the human body outlives its joints, its cognitive and memory capacities, it does not mean that we have to take it for granted that neurologic diseases and dementias are identical with old age. Ageing is essentially historical. This means that what happens in advanced age cannot be seen quite independently from what happens during the whole life. Coping with functional limitation is connected with the ability to carve out meaningful roles for every situation of our life.

To Know The Self Includes to Know The Body

Most of us consider health as one of the most desirable and important values of our lives. Health is often valued only in its absence. It may also be seen as a means to other valued ends, and not as an end in itself. The literature over the past thirty years shows the difficulties of a definition of health. Nevertheless, nearly all broad definitions of health echo the classical models of health as harmony among the body's processes, or the concept of disease as disturbance of equilibrium (Blaxter 1995: 2).

It is a matter of individual responsibility to chose the method of administrating the lifestyle according to one's values. But anyhow, cultivating awareness, learning to cope with emotions, training harmonious integration of mind and body are efforts which most of us would consider as important activities for achieving health and well-being.

Although in our Western tradition these attitudes are highly estimated, their moral meaning and not their curative value has always been considered. It is in oriental cultures that we find systematic teaching practicing such attitudes for the sake of mental and physical health.

The psychiatrist and philosopher, Karl Jaspers, was the first to direct attention towards oriental methods as conducive to mental health (Jaspers 1948). Jaspers saw that meditation includes scientifically valid elements, meaningful in therapy as self-control, allowing a person to change his mental attitudes by means of his own strength. According to Tomio Hirai, who has been very influenced by the philosophy of Jaspers, the practice of meditation regulates the operation of the autonomous system and eliminates tensions that affect the cerebral cortex. In this way it brings stability to the spirit and returns health to the body. This is the scientific corroboration for oriental philosophy that the mind and the body are one (Hirai 1978).

What is common to Selye's stress theory and oriental philosophical and medical ideas, is the conviction that to know the self has an inherent curative value and that to know the self includes to know the body (Selye 1975: 406). The only way to conduct and know the body is through feeling. Awareness begins with the sensations of the processes of our body. At every moment our bodies go through physiological and psychological changes of which we are unaware; but when we are conscious of these changes, we can more easily cope with our difficulties. When our awareness is undeveloped, our senses do not register the impressions received. In order to develop higher awareness, we need to integrate body and mind. Whenever we are sick, unbalanced, or have negative feelings, we feel the isolated organ or unrelated symptoms like some alien quality in ourselves. In order to be heathy we should learn how to balance body and mind. As we know, our bodies and minds have the resources to protect themselves. The cure for sickness is within us if we bring ourselves back into balance so that the energy is flowing smoothly. According to Selye we must try to attain the great art to express our vitality through the particular channels and at the particular speed which nature foresaw for us (Selye 1975: 419).

According to oriental philosophy we can cultivate the healing energy within our feeling through relaxation. If our muscles work well together, free from superfluous tension, then we will have the concentration necessary for full experience. Through relaxation we discover a new way of integration of body, mind and environment; the key lies within our feelings and sensations. Through relaxation, we awaken these feelings which then expand and accumulate (Tulku 1977).

In short, according to modern physiology self-knowledge and self-cure are possible, but the methods to achieve this aim are those of oriental cultures. Scientific physiology shows that body processes can be changed by conscious activity but traditionally it is expected that the influence must be a causal relationship. Oriental methods show that the interrelation between the self and the body processes is much more complicated than the causal relationship. For example, the practice of meditation relaxes tension that affects the cerebral cortex and in this way it can bring stability to the spirit and health to the body. From the viewpoint of modern neurophysiology this can mean devising a way to convert tense beta brain waves into the alpha or theta waves which are the usual state of the brain of a person in a calm and relaxed situation (Hirai 1978: 64). Now the method of achieving this aim, as we know, is mainly concentration and control of thought, which means thinking of nothing. On the other hand, the way to develop control of the mind and to cultivate the power to concentrate is to be interested in many things and to be receptive to many different kinds of stimuli (Hirai 1978: 73).

Perhaps if we better understand both scientific physiology and oriental methods of self-care, we will not always need to depend on external and artificial means to stay healthy and free from pain.

References

Blaxter, M.
  1995   *Health and Lifestyles*, Tavistock: London/New York.

Canguilhelm, George
  1972   *Le normal et le pathologique*, Presses Universitaires de France: Paris.

Cannon, Walter
  1947   *The Wisdom of the Body*, Kegan Paul, Trench, Trubner & Co.: London.

Davison, Charlie & Davey Smith, George
  1995   "The baby and the bath water: examining socio-cultural and free-market critiques of health promotion", in: R. Bunton, S. Nettleton and R. Burrows (eds.): *The Sociology of Health Promotion: Critical Analysis of Consumption, Lifestyle and Risk*, pp. 91-99, Routledge: London/New York.

Descartes, René
  1984   *Les Passions de l'àme*, French/German, K. Hammacher (ed. translation), Mainer: Hamburg.

Hepworth, Mike
  1995   "Positive ageing: what is the message?", in: R. Bunton, S. Nettleton and R. Burrows (eds.): *The Sociology of Health Promotion: Critical Analyses of Consumption, Lifestyle and Risk*, pp. 176-190, Routledge: London/New York.

Hirai, Tomio
  1978   *Zen and the Mind: Scientific Approach to Zen Practice*, Japan Publications: Tokyo.

Jaspers, Karl
  1948   *Allgemeine Psychopathologie*, Springer: Berlin/Heidelberg.

Reesor, Margaret
  1989   *The Nature of Man in Early Stoic Philosophy*, Duckworth: London.

Selye, Hans
1975 *The Stress of Life*, McGraw-Hill Book Company: New York/London/Toronto.

Tsouyopoulos, Nelly
1988 "The Mind-Body Problem in Medicine: The Crisis of Medical Anthropology and its Historical Preconditions", in: *Hist. Phil. Life Sci.* (10 Suppl.): 55-74.

Tulku, Tartan
1977 *Gesture of Balance: A Guide to Awareness, Self-healing and Meditation*, Dharma Publishing: Berkeley CA.

Lifestyle, Charismatic Ideology and a Praxis Aesthetic

by David Aldridge

"A pure aesthetic expresses, in rationalized form, the ethos of a cultured elite or, in other words, of the dominated fraction of the dominant class. As such, it is a misrecognized social relationship. 'The denial of lower, coarse, vulgar, venal, servile – in a word, natural – enjoyment, which constitutes the sacred sphere of culture, implies an affirmation of the superiority of those who can be satisfied with the sublimated, refined, disinterested, gratuitous, distinguished pleasures forever closed to the profane. That is why art and cultural consumption are predisposed, consciously, and deliberately or not, to fulfil a social function of legitimating social differences'" (Randal Johnson quoting Pierre Bourdieu 1993: 25).

The main impulse for this paper came to me from a variety of sources. These sources are incidents taken from daily life and, although they are anecdotal, they indicate the difficulties that we face when we talk about health and the practices that are used to maintain and promote such health. Indeed, one of the significant points of this paper will be that health is heterogeneous and that such ideas come out of the practice of daily living rather than being homogenous and based upon a rationalist unified theory. Such a demand for consistency may be misleading (Kirmayer 1994) and hide the discrepancies between varying forms of knowledge. While the above quote is made with regard to art and literature as cultural processes, I shall be arguing that health too is a cultural process and can be similarly subjected to an aesthetic critique.

I want to use a few introductory anecdotes for two reasons. First, we see how health is a complex set of ideas, and secondly, that we need to consider the day-to-day narratives of individuals as they talk about health. This latter point is not new in terms of heath-care research and qualitative methods (Milburn 1996; Radley & Billig 1996), but what I will also be suggesting is that most research makes an assumption that health and illness are opposing poles of a continuum. My proposal is that health and illness may be so constructed by health-care professionals trained to think in such a way, but such an ideology may not be reflected in the everyday lives of other people. Perhaps the realms of health and illness are quite separate in practice? Rather than being oppositional they are competing discourses (McRobbie 1996) relevant for making sense of particular situations.

The first incident is one that occurred at one of the Copenhagen meetings: Following the usual presentations about health and various approaches to medicine, we duly retired to eat and then to the bar, where several colleagues ordered their drinks and smoked cigarettes. For most of the day we had been sitting in a centrally heated room and had taken part in no strenuous activities other than disagreeing with each other in a mild sort of way and occasionally moving our chairs to let others get by. From some perspectives of health-care activity, we were behaving quite irresponsibly; smoking, drinking both coffee and alcohol, pursuing sedentary activities and no doubt eating fatty foods. However, those of us partaking in such activities seemed to be paying little attention to "health" as such and were generally getting on with the day-to-day business of living, part of which was actively pleasurable. As such this is a rejection of an aesthetics of Kantian 'pure' taste and an embracing of a Bourdieuian 'vulgar' taste that returns to the senses. And it is this notion of sensuousness that is at the heart of the original meaning of aesthetic in that it springs from the lower animal passions, a matter of literal taste.

One of the burdens, or joys, of being a conference delegate is that one has to take part in social activities. It so happened that I was invited to the German beer festival in Munich, and not wanting to offend my hosts, I duly took part. The festival takes place in a huge park complete with fairground activities that are replete with noise and activity, and charged with the electricity of human beings having fun. Within the festival grounds there are huge barns where people go to be entertained. The group I was with were duly led to such a barn and as the doors opened I was immediately reminded of many of the things my mother had told me not to do as a boy and which seemed enjoyable as a man. From out of the open doors came a billow of smoke, gales of laughter, squalls of music from a German "oompah" band and the wonderful breezy beery odours of the hall. All the perils of enjoyment captured together in a storm of experience. It will be my own fault if I do not make it to old age. And here lies the crux of the argument, most of the health-care debates are moralistic and ignore a profound factor in human existence, repeated from the first example, and that is the simple activity of pleasure.

Another scene occurred in a restaurant. My wife and I had decided to take an early Spring walk, the weather was fine and after a gentle stroll we arrived at a hotel in time for lunch, as planned I might add. During the meal, a number of middle-aged women came to sit at the next table. The first topic of conversation was their health and each woman took turns to talk about her current ailments. In doing so she introduced various connected topics like the state of her family, the well-being of her husband, the relative benefits of being mature, where she had been shopping recently and a general philosophy and outlook on life. While we might as professionals be tempted to look at this as a health-care narrative, health being the chosen topic of introduction, we would be missing a valuable point. Health was used as a springboard for a widely ranging conversation that did not itself remain focused on health. As the stereotypical greeting "Hello, how are you?" rarely intends to elicit a conversation about the person's state of health, health as a subject of naturally occurring narratives plays only a minor role. All too often we consider health as if it were the peak of a unified pyramid of rational consonant understandings, rather than a topic in a constellation of understandings some of which may be dissonant. It is knowing the relationships between elements of such a constellation that might help us to understand health as part of daily living, as praxis.

When I was a small boy my grandfather took me to the local park where he sat with his cronies, and I played. To give himself some respite from me, he would suggest that I ran around the bowling green. He would either time me, to see how fast I could run, or he would count how many times I had completed the circuit. This was play and I would imagine myself to be some athletic hero of the day like Chris Brasher or Emil Zatopek. Such play became a sport as I grew up and started cross-country running. In my twenties I played other sports and ran, not only for the simple fun of it, but because I wanted to improve my fitness. Fitness to play sport, that is, not as a health activity. In my thirties, I started to study again and as an aid to preparing for my examinations began to run every day after studying. In my forties, my father had his first heart attack and I began running again, not for enjoyment this time, but as a hedge against angina. However, I soon stopped as there was no pleasure in such activity and I was picking up more minor injuries "jogging" than going for my daily walk. If we take the same activity, in this case running, we can infer differing attributes to it and the benefits that it may have brought for my health. Biddle (1995) refers to this as the "feel good factor". Indeed, people had seen my running in my thirties and thought I was doing it for my health. This was quite false. I did it for the sheer pleasure of running like a boy and as a practical activity that would enable me to enjoy playing. Only later did the same activity gain overtones of a health-care activity. It is precisely this aspect of understanding such an activity in relationship to a broader field of understandings and activities that is important.

As a final example I would like to refer again to the element of pleasure and how it is ignored in health-care thinking. A current debate has been about the implication of cholesterol in coronary heart disease (Evans, Barer, & Marmor 1994) where eating a fatty diet is seen to be unhealthy behaviour. A favourable way of eating has been proposed as the "Mediterranean diet" that includes less fats, less meat, more fruit and vegetables and carbohydrate like breads and pastas. Again, in the spirit of academic benevolence, I have eaten in the Mediterranean and holidayed on a Greek island. Apart from the incidence of cigarette smoking that accompanied such meals, there were several cultural factors rarely mentioned in health-care directives about diet that might play a significant role. First, the meals were slow affairs often partaken within a large family group that occurred late in the evening. Cultural setting seems to be conveniently forgotten in health-care descriptions of diet. Second, the food was enjoyed as an activity amongst a series of activities which might include dancing or going for a stroll outside to take the evening air. Yet the palpable enjoyment of the food as an eating activity and as a social occasion had little to do with the seeming narrow aspect of nutrition. Perhaps the reason for the failing inducements to change dietary habits (Meillier, Lund, & Kok 1996; Nguyen, Otis, & Potvin 1996) are simply that such inducements demonstrate a poverty of understanding concerning the human activity of eating together as a pleasurable activity and the previously mentioned constellation of activities that make health part of a complex praxis aesthetic. Hamilton et al (1995) refer to vegetarians as eating from a moral menu, and it is this virtuous aspect of acceptable conduct that appears to pervade health-care arguments. The dispute of the primacy of reason over sensuousness is not a new argument in European thought and appears also to have ramifications in Chinese political thinking (Gu 1996).

Health as Identity

In modern times, health is no longer a state of not being sick. Individuals are choosing to become healthy and, in some cases, declare themselves as pursuing the activity of being well. This change, from attributing the status *"being sick"* to engaging in the activity of "becoming well", is a reflection of a modern trend whereby individuals are taking the definition of themselves into their own hands rather than relying upon an identity being imposed by another. Being recognized as a "healthy" person is, for some, an important feature of a modern identity. While personal active involvement has always been present in health-care maintenance and prevention, in that people have strategies of distress management (Aldridge 1994), a new development appears to be that being a *"healthy"*, *"creative"*, *"musical"* or *"spiritual"* person is considered to be significant in the composition of an individual's *"lifestyle"*. Rather than strategies of personal health management in response to sickness, we see an *assemblage* of activities designed to promote health and prevent sickness. These activities are incorporated under the rubric of *"lifestyle"* and sometimes refer to the pursuit of "emotional wellbeing" (Furnham 1994). Furthermore, such a lifestyle is intimately bound up with how a person chooses to define him- or herself.

Thus, I am arguing here that postmodern identities are constructed, and although these identities are bound up with cultural values, they focus primarily on the body. What we need to take heed of as health-care professionals is that this *"body work"*, this embodiment of culture (Kirmayer 1994; Lewis 1995; Starrett 1995; Turner 1995), this corporeality of expression, is a pleasurable activity, often recreational and simply not medical. Bodies are done, they become the material aspect of both the individual and the culture in which he or she is embodied. The presentation of symptoms by a patient, for example, has an articulacy that is based upon the body and its needs. The naming by the medical practitioner of the entities to which those symptoms refer is based upon a different articulacy that is based in language and reason. The somatic has an aesthetic based upon the senses, while diagnosis has an ethic based upon naming (Khushf 1996). For the patient, the process of naming, putting words to a private somatic sensation and communicating that sensation within a context of reason, the medical encounter, changes the experience of that sensation (Cioffi 1996).

The definition of health, who is to define what health is, and who is to be involved in healing, are not new activities. Such issues are raised at times of transformation, when the old order is being challenged (Aldridge 1991). In postmodern society, orthodoxies are challenged, and as truth is regarded as relative with few fixed authorities to turn to, identities can be composed from a palette of cultural alternatives.

Health is also appearing in modern society as a commodity. Far from being a simple object, health is concerned with social relationships representing personal worth, market values, existential principles and theological niceties. However, the location of health in modern terms is often within the body (Charmaz 1995; Kelly & Field 1996; Wallulis 1994). People are demanding recognition that they play an active role in their own health-care, and that some can act as lay health-care practitioners. Indeed, before we ask a doctor or any licensed practitioner, we have been through varying cycles of self-care, asking family and friends or just hoping that the problem will go away. This shift away from authority and orthodoxy towards democratisation and choice reflects a change from a belief in the certainties of science and religion to a relativist position where people literally "make up" their own minds and work on their bodies; that is, we construct our own identities.

As a consequence of challenges to traditional authority, and the collapse of state socialism here in Europe, there is no longer a possibility for some individuals to relate to a given social order. In the writings of many health-care practitioners, particularly in alternative medicine, there are few references to health care as being a social product for the benefit of communities. Instead, rather than a communal argument being voiced, there appears to be an argument for the individual located in an ecological context; the "green" politics of environmental liberalism. Such a perspective ignores the notion of population and health and the pervading fact that morbidity is correlated with the distribution of wealth (Evans, Barer, & Marmor 1994; Vågerö 1994).

Individuals are seeking to treat themselves with a long-term eclectic health strategy that includes a palette of activities with the support of chosen, albeit diverse, informed advisers who can fulfil the role of facilitator. Health-care consumers are blurring the role between the traditional health-care services delivered at times of crisis, with those of preventive strategies based on consumerism. The idea of community health in these descriptions may be alluded to as an ecological context, but there is little reference to an immediate social or communal context. This is a reflection of the Romantic notion of the individual related directly with the cosmos (Tsouyopoulos 1984).

Medicines as Charismatic Ideologies

My principal criticism of health-care arguments as presented by conventional medicine, and many complementary medical initiatives, is that these approaches are founded upon a charismatic ideology; that is, health is pursued for health's sake. While this may be relevant for religion – life for a divine being's sake –, or for art – art for art's sake –, health will always be undermined by the reality of the body. Health, religion and art are presented as metaphysical activities – they are above the physical realm. But, like the body of work in terms of art products, the individual body in terms of physical health is subject to temporality and is not above the substantial plane of existence. Health is temporal and locally corporeal. We may be better advised to defer from the charismatic ideology of "C" medicines; that is, conventional and complementary, and seek a functional aesthetic relating to the performed body. To be accepted as a performance, a *habitus* (Bourdieu 1993), there must be an audience and that returns us to a cultural and social field.

While body size and shape are aspects of personal identity, it is how the body is interpreted, the aesthetics of health beliefs that play an important role in forming identity. Such beliefs play an active part in how we recognize illness and what therapy form we choose (Aldridge 1992). Meanings provide a bridge between cultural and physiological phenomena. The diagnosis of a medical complaint is also a statement about personal identity (Stravynski & O'Connor 1995; van der Geest 1994) and the stigma that may be attached to such an identity (Crossley 1995). Symbolic meanings are the loci of power whereby illness is explained and controlled. Such loci are now shifting from the educated health professionals, to the increasingly better-educated, and health-conscious, consumers although that relationship is delicate (Dickinson 1995).

Indeed, in the postmodern era there are ever increasing producers of symbolic goods as related to health. Various agencies, including consumer groups, now make claims for cultural legitimacy in competition with the orthodoxies of conventional medicine (although it appears sometimes that complementary medical agencies have been incorporated within the body of conventionality). The notion of alternative medicine, consumer groups and self-care groups have struggled to liberate health from the grip of academic control and the monolith of conventional medicine. This has been linked to the development of individual autonomy whereby the health of the individual can be performed as he or she sees fit. Health has the potential of a style and form liberated from a subordination to political and medical interests. To paraphrase Bourdieu:

> "The mass production of works produced by quasi-industrial methods – coincided with the extension of the public, resulting from the expansion of primary education, which turned new classes (including women) into consumers of culture. The development of the system of cultural production is accompanied by a process of differentiation generated by the diversity of the publics at which the different categories of producers aim their products" (Bourdieu 1993: 113).

Definition of Health in a Cultural Context

It is clear that in our modern cultures several belief systems operate in parallel and can coexist. Patients have begun to demand that their understandings about health play a role in their care, and practitioners too are seeking complementary understandings. Health itself is a state subject to social and individual definition. What counts as healthy is dependent upon cultural norms. Health and disease are not fixed entities but concepts used to characterise a process of adaptation to meet the changing demands of life and the changing *meanings* given to living. Negotiating what counts as healthy is a process we are all involved in, as are the forms of treatment, welfare and care which we choose to accept as adequate or satisfactory (Aldridge 1990, Santiago-Izarry 1996).

Spickard (1994), in an earlier volume, reminded us that modern people do not merely accept the identities passed down by authorities. Instead, they construct their identities from various sources. Modern identity is eclectic. As in the age of Romanticism, when revolution demanded a new way of being, the primacy of the perceiver is once more being emphasized. Subjectivity becomes paramount, on the one hand reifying the individual, but on the other hand running the risk that the individual will become isolated. Indeed, while post-modernism is perhaps itself characterised by a revolt against authority and tends towards self-referentiality, its very eclecticism leaves the individual valued but exhausted by significance – what Gergen (1991) refers to as "the saturated self". This move towards the ability of the individual to control her- or himself has led Pinell (1996) to refer to the *homo medicus*, the sick person who objectifies her- or himself as a medical auxiliary.

Brewster Smith (1994) suggests that the inflated potential for selfhood dislocated from traditional value sources increases the potential for despair, and while individuals may rise to the challenge of pluralism, there are some individuals who will seek to join groups that offer some form of reassurance in a given orthodoxy of beliefs and actions. The danger in modern Europe is that the romantic notion of individualism becomes perverted into nationalism, and the dislocated individual seeking to construct his or her own identity joins a group intent on the limitation of others' freedom of self-definition whereby he or she can maintain their security. Consensus is fragile in a context where individual demands are reified.

If the self in modern society is always being constructed to meet the variety of life's contingencies, then we move away from the model of one generation initiating the next generation into the truths of its own beliefs. Instead, there is a pool of experts and advisers to whom we can turn when constructing a system of beliefs within a cultural ecology – ecological, in the sense that those beliefs are connected, and that the consequences of those beliefs, when acted out in the real world, are related one to another. In some modern alternative healing approaches, traditional forms of teaching by initiation and learning by discipline are rejected in favour of an eclecticism that takes techniques and locates them within a culture of meanings improvised according to the situation. This action itself is political. Rejecting given orthodoxies, and demanding freedom to engage in the project of realising one's "self" is a *"politics of life-decisions concerning life-styles"* (Brewster Smith 1994). And as Hughes (1996) suggests, a performative and dramatic approach overrides both traditional and deconstructive notions of causality.

Health as Functional Aesthetic

The notion of lifestyle appears to be important in describing modern approaches to health-care use and its delivery. In a Foucaultian sense, the self is not an assemblage of functional components, but a unified style of behaviour (Dreyfus 1987). However, I am challenging such a perspective in this paper. Rather than there being a human nature, the self-interpreting practice of being human enables us to have varying natures. Our lives have the potential to become a work of art in that our identities are constructed and maintained each day (Aldridge 1989), thus, a performed identity and a functional aesthetic. In this sense the activity of healing is concerned not with restricting us to a one-dimensional sense of being according to an accepted orthodox world view, but the possibility for the interpretation of the self as new albeit embedded as an identity within a particular culture.

Individuals then seek to make claims about their personal identity to someone else to whom they matter; that is, in interaction. Claiming to be a healthy, fulfilled, empowered, artistic or spiritual person, is a way of presenting self that will elicit a response from others. Schwalbe (1993) interprets this action of deciding which identity to present, and how we present ourselves, as one of moral agency. In modern descriptions of alternative healing, it is the body that is the stage for the interaction of the self and its interaction with culture.

If the big narratives of modernism are now being replaced by our own personal sets of meaning made locally with those with whom we seek to live (Warde 1994), then we need to understand more about the person that sits before us in our consulting room. How that person creates an identity will be indicative of how that person will resolve his or her problems. How that person seeks to be identified will guide his or her health-care activities. Some will seek medications, others will imbibe herbal preparations, others will seek to be physically manipulated, others will seek to be psychically manipulated, yet others will exchange energies both subtle and cosmic, some will search for the laying on of hands in a ritual way – whether it be from a medical doctor or a spiritual healer (both require their own brands of faith) – some will sing to relieve their souls, and others will jog for their hearts' content. Each of these, the bodybuilder and the disciple, the artist and the atheist, the athlete and the allopath, will demand recognition for whom they are as a person, and for that recognition to be included in treatment decisions. Indeed, the route to treatment will be guided by an itinerary pertinent to personal identity. Health is something that is done, a performed art.

What we singularly fail to see is that our current thinking about health is dominated by a medical thinking that ignores much of the reality of the persons we intend to treat and support. Few people, when they are sick, respond by seeking a health-care practitioner (Andersen 1996). Perhaps even fewer consult a health-care practitioner about staying healthy. What we appear to do, outside of an academic life thinking about such lofty matters, is eat, drink, amuse ourselves, love our nearest and dearest, walk the dog, chase pieces of leather across a field (both dogs and football players), without thinking of medical consequences. Maybe our health-care assumptions are so narrow that they have little relevance for others who do not bow down at the altars of epidemiology and empiricism. Many lay appraisals of health-care activity seem to be based upon holistic considerations that include feelings of mood and vitality (Andersen & Lobel 1995). If changes of mood are ignored, or assessed as potentially pathological by health-care practitioners, and the philosophy of vitality is generally regarded as invalid in modern scientific medicine, then we should not wonder that few people come to us for help. If, as in traditional Chinese medicine, for example, health seeking becomes a pleasure that sequesters " *a body that can not only taste sweetness but be sweet, not only report painful symptoms, but also dwell on and cultivate the quiet comforts of health*" (Farquhar 1994: 493) then maybe we can understand that the seeking of a positive identity in a postmodern world is an activity that can be enjoyed without experts and the grand narratives of science and medicine. We may indeed have to learn to seek out those personal and local truths that our patients are themselves choosing to embody.

It may appear that self and society are being presented as opposing realities. However, in the field of health promotion we know that to choose only one approach would be limited. In this century, major changes in health status have occurred as results of improvements in living conditions – clean water, improved sanitation and adequate nutrition. There is also evidence that income plays an important role in maintaining standards of health, that poverty is not only a social burden; for the individual it has consequences for personal health. The field of health influences as they are played out in the community manifest themselves in the bodies of individual persons.

In the last decade of the twentieth century there is a change in relationship between self and society. The individual is becoming disembedded from a traditional commitment to society, a disenchantment with the collective, and a new type of commitment is being seen (Warde 1994). In a liberal ideology, individuals with enough disposable income are becoming personally responsible for their own identity and this is linked to lifestyle as commodity. Individuals are socialised in a postmodern society as consumers with a choice of lifestyles. While on the one hand our autonomy is restricted in the field of employment (if we can find employment), how we choose to define ourselves and with whom we choose to define ourselves is a matter of personal freedom. An anomaly of this situation is that personal perceptions of health, own wellbeing and life satisfaction may be at odds with a health professional's assessment of that individual's health status (Albrecht 1994). The danger of this individual health lifestyle approach, when it assumes that health is the opposing pole of a health-illness construct, is that individuals too can be held responsible for the causation of their own diseases (Kirkwood & Brown 1995) and lifestyle factors can be seen as the precursors, risk factors, of future illness (Armstrong 1995). Health may then become expressed as a moral debate concerning responsible citizens free from the intervention of doctors. This in turn masks the agenda of restricting access to limited resources. Rather than the sick being labelled as deviant, the sick become labelled as illegitimate users of provisions. In England such a situation has occurred whereby advertisements in national newspapers have been taken out on behalf of a medical association requesting patients only to contact their doctor in an emergency.

Promoting and maintaining our health is one such choice in the plethora of consumer activities intimately related to our identity. The bodybuilder, eating efficiently for the production of a body mass, will consume differently from the computer freak who surfs the Internet and eats fast food for a fast lifestyle. Both these will differ from the jogging yoghurt eater who consumes vegetables to purify his material self and reduce his cholesterol levels, and meditates for the salvation of the planet. The young boy who was running for fun in my earlier example, grew up to be the young man running for pleasure, who became the middle-aged man running for his life. While the same activity prevailed through each episode, the needs that were being gratified were different (see also Montelpare & Kanters 1994; Tinsley & Eldredge 1995).

The implication of Bourdieu's work (see Randal Johnson in Bourdieu 1993) is that any analysis that overlooks the social grounds of aesthetic taste tends to establish a universal aesthetic and cultural practices that are in fact products of privilege. So it is of an universal health practice. A pure aesthetic demands keeping necessity at arms length, and daily life will always subvert such a health aesthetic, thus my call for a functional aesthetic of health understandings based upon the body, that legitimates pleasure. Martin (1996: 53) urges us to an *"understanding of the imagery, language and metaphor operating in our contemporary culture of the body"*.

Implications for Health Promotion

I would like to consider three practical areas of health-care that relate to the previous arguments. All are subject to the charismatic ideology that assumes a monolithic perspective on health as applied by experts who know that it is often based upon a hidden moral agenda.

The first is concerned with AIDS educational campaigns that are concerned with encouraging safe sex amongst gay men. Such educational material has assumed that there is an homogenous culture to which gay men belong, and that behaviourial change will follow as a logical consequence from reasoned exhortation. Gold argues otherwise (1995). There is not a safe sex culture in existence, and the encouragement to have safe sex has missed out on the reality of hedonism involved in sexual contact. As mentioned previously, health-care rationale, for the individual, is not necessarily linked to a carefully planned strategy as health-care professionals like to believe. There may be indeed disparities between what people believe and what they do.

For some gay men, the constellation of sexual gratification, recreational pleasure and the maintenance of a particular lifestyle, tied up as it is with a gay identity, does not have health-care as a principal strategy for living, even in a climate of AIDS prevention. Human beings live, with optimism and zest, to enjoy life, not necessarily to prevent illness. Any interventions aimed at changing behaviour in gay men to promote a safer sex culture will need to acccpt that there are groups of men with differing lifestyles and expectations, some of whom may not be benign and benevolent towards a wider community.

A second example is in the field of dieting and exercise as they are related to body shape. Females in Western industrialised cultures are expressing not only concern about their bodily shapes but are actively engaged in altering how they appear. The female body is the interface between the woman herself, as a person, and her social identity. Feelings about the self are related to feelings about the body; they are not solely located in the body, but are concerned with how that body appears to others. A vast amount of time and money are spent on consumer activities related to this body image in terms of exercise activities, fashion and diet. Slimness has become popularly associated with elegance, self-control, social attractiveness and youth (Furnham, Titman, & Sleeman 1994). Such descriptions are also the motivating factors associated with the sales pitch of many consumer products. While such personal lifestyles of dieting for fitness and the presentation of a powerful potent body may be health enabling, there is also the paradox that it is these very activities that are involved in the generation of eating disorders. Hartley (1996) argues that the advancement of health education encouraging a diet low in fat and cholesterol has a negative effect and may play a role in eating disorders. The aesthetic of near emaciation in conjunction with the modern moral imperative of eating healthily, that is fat-free, may encourage a lifestyle that is life threatening. Health promotion has a social ecology that is all too easily neglected and this neglect of context may be the cause of high relapse rates following health promotion interventions (Stokols et al 1996).

The encouragement of excessive individualism, while promoting autonomy, may be at the expense of a woman's integrity as a whole person. She is connected to a set of cultural values that threaten to destroy her health when disembedded from the relations that may offer a social meaning to her personal identity. This excessive emphasis on the individual body dislocated from the social body is classically reflected in the egoism explanation in Durkheim's explanation of suicide (Warde 1994). Food preparation, the choosing of diet, the presentation of the body and the adornment of the body are never fixed and belong to a complex argument related both to individual identity and to the maintenance of a symbolic capital (Rasmussen 1996).

A third example is concerned with cigarette smoking in the young. While there has been a considerable impact on behalf of educational campaigns to curb adult smoking, those campaigns have failed to make any impact on the prevalence of young smokers (Lynch 1995). Lynch argues that this failure is because educational campaigns singularly fail to understand the reasons why young people smoke. These reasons may not be homogenous, and certainly will not follow the causal sensible logic of most health-care professionals. Image is seen as a powerful factor in influencing smoking behaviour, as is the need to be "an individual". Thus, campaigns aimed to curb enjoyment, emphasizing a sensible conformity to an artificially constructed target group of adolescent smokers falsely assumed to be homogenous, will be doomed to failure.

We see that hedonism, the enjoyment of the body, the maintenance of a self-image and pursuing an active, seemingly healthy, lifestyle can be both health promoting but in some circumstances deleterious to health. The pursuit of excessive individualism may lead to a disentanglement from social relationships that are vital to bringing some checks and balances to counter extremes of living that may prove to be deleterious. There is no easy reconciliation of this problem.

We must, however, recognize that our health-care endeavours must target small groups and individuals. There are no easy global solutions that can be applied from the top-down. Struggling to understand the individual and those with whom she is bound are vital. If this is central to the practice of health-care in the consulting room, then it can surely be extended to our health-care reasoning.

The ramification of all this for health-care is that instead of a top-down approach to promoting health-care, we must consider targeting interventions aimed at small groups in which individuals are embedded. Even within church groups we know there are small groups of individuals who have differing interpretations and adopt differing lifestyles (Spickard 1994).

We have to understand how people "do" their lives, not simply what they think and say about their lives. It is in the body that individual identity is expressed, and the body is the interface between the individual and society. It is what people do together that binds them together with the groups with whom they perform their lives. This performance will be bound up with lifestyle, exercise and leisure activities (Johnson, Boyle & Heller 1995; Montelpare & Kanters 1994; Tinsley & Eldredge 1995), home decoration (Madigan & Munro 1996), dieting (Furnham & Boughton 1995; Hamilton et al 1995; Nguyen, Otis & Potvin 1996) and dress. In this sense, "lifestyle" is not something that can be read about in books; it is an activity and also subject to change (Træen 1995). Making sense of the world is an activity achieved through the body. Swimming cannot be learned about by reading about it, or by gathering together a band of expert swimmers to tell you about their experiences, nor by attending a conference of hydro-physicists. At some time we have to jump into the water and through experience do it. The body grasps what it needs to do. Having a teacher in the water certainly helps. So too with health and a change in "lifestyle". If we wish to encourage people to do something differently, we have to understand that it will be intimately connected with their identity as a person and those with whom that identity is validated. Health-care professionals are no longer the group with whom our patients wish to identify, and with their rates of suicide, marital disruption and drug abuse, who can blame them. Change is brought about by influencing small groups and understanding their way of being in the world.

One factor that we must take into account is that the serious business of living can also be fun. While we know a lot about health-care activities and their impact, we know little about the importance of leisure activities and their ramifications for health. Positive emotions, according to new thinking, influence our health status for the better. Optimism and a sensual pleasure in everyday activities and situations are valuable for promoting personal health and the absence of symptoms and a sense of enjoyment coupled with a zest for living, appear to play a significant role in the subjective assessment of health (Montelpare & Kanters 1994; Wenglert & Rosén 1995). Once more, health is an activity that has sensual ramifications that are also concerned with pleasurable activities that are themselves integrated with an overall sense of "lifestyle" rather than our unilateral exhortations to follow health-care prescriptions.

How such optimism and sensual pleasure is passed on to those living in poverty as the urban poor will be the proving ground of the post-modernist argument and its reification of individualism. That the poor may continue to smoke and drink as creature comforts in a harsh world may lend credibility to the argument that sensual pleasures and leisure activities, even when there is no work, are the important arbiters of health-care activity as it relates to daily living. The distribution of wealth that has a considerable impact of morbidity is not in the hands of individuals but belongs to a broader political process.

At the beginning of this chapter I used a quote from Pierre Bourdieu that separates the pure aesthetic of a dominant class from that of natural vulgar enjoyment. The same situation occurs in the broader medical discourse, whether it be within the supremacist dogma of orthodox medicine, or the moral stricture of complementary medicine as they have both become established in modern Western health-care delivery. There is a pure aesthetic of health related to a dominant moral discourse. What I am arguing for is a vulgar praxis aesthetic that takes health as being done. This reflects both the chthonian mode of knowing – touch and smell – with the Apollonian mode – seeing and being seen (Bemporad 1996). Rather than separating forms of knowing, perhaps we can turn to a reconciliation that occurs in the practice of everyday life. The body that is done is both seen and smelt in practice. Health-care understandings are then heterogeneous, combining both sense and reason located in the practice of everyday living. This will have an implication for the methodologies that we use for health-care research as we need to incorporate – literally embody – lay knowledge (Aldridge 1990, 1992; Emke 1996; Popay and Williams 1996).

References

Albrecht, Gary
    1994   "Subjective health assessment", in: C. Jenkinson (ed.): *Measuring health and medical outcomes*, UCL Press: London.

Aldridge, David
    1989   "A phenomenological comparison of the organization of music and the self", in: *Arts in Psychotherapy*, 16: 91-97.
    1990   "Making and taking health care decisions", in: *Journal of the Royal Society of Medicine*, 83: 720-723.
    1991   "Healing and medicine", in: *Journal of the Royal Society of Medicine*, 84: 516-518.
    1992   "The needs of individual patients in clinical research", in: *Advances*, 8: 58-65.
    1994   "Unconventional medicine in Europe", in: *Advances*, 10: 52-60.

Andersen, Jørgen Ø.
    1996   "Lifestyles, Consumption and Alternative Therapies", this volume.

Andersen, Marin & Lobel, Marci
    1995   "Predictors of health self-appraisal: what's involved in feeling healthy?", in: *Basic and Applied Social Psychology*, 16: 121-136.

Armstrong, David
1995 "The rise of surveillance medicine", in: *Sociology of Health and Illness,* 17: 393-404.

Bemporad, Jules
1996 "Selfstarvation through the ages: Reflections on the pre-history of anorexia nervosa", in: *International Journal of Eating Disorders*, 19(3): 217-237.

Biddle, Stuart
1995 "Exercise and social health", in: *Research Quarterly for Exercise and Sport,* 66: 292-297.

Bourdieu, Pierre
1993 *The field of cultural production,* Columbia University Press: New York.

Brewster Smith, M.
1994 "Selfhood at risk: postmodern perils and the perils of postmodernism", in: *American Psychologist,* 49: 405-411.

Charmaz, Kathy
1995 "The body, identity, and self: Adapting to impairment", in: *The Sociological Quarterly,* 36: 657-680.

Cioffi, Delia
1996 "Making public the private: Possible effects of expressing somatic experience", in: *Psychology and Health,* 11: 203-222.

Crossley, Nick
1995 "Body techniques, agency and intercorporeality: On Goffman's relations in public", in: *Sociology,* 29: 133-149.

Dickinson, Roger
1995 "Two cultures – one voice? Problems in broadcaster/health educator co-operation", in: *Health Education Research,* 10: 421-430.

Dreyfus, Hubert
1987 "Foucault's critique of psychiatric medicine", in: *The Journal of Medicine and Philosophy,* 12: 311-333.

Emke, Ivan
1996 "Methodology and methodolatry: Creativity and the improvishment of the imagination in sociology", in: *Canadian Journal of Sociology,* 21(1): 77-90.

Evans, Robert, Barer, Morris and Marmor, Theodore
1994 *Why are some people healthy and others not?* Aldine de Gruyter: New York.

Farquhar, Judith
1994 "Eating Chinese medicine", in: *Cultural Anthropology,* 9: 471-497.

Furnham, Adrian
1994 "Explaining health and illness: lay perceptions on current and future health, the causes of illness and the nature of recovery", in: *Social Science and Medicine,* 39: 715-725.

Furnham, Adrian and Boughton, Joanne
1995 "Eating behaviour and body dissatisfaction among dieters, aerobic exercisers and a control group", in: *European Eating Disorders Review,* 3: 35-45.

Furnham, Adrian, Titman, Penny and Sleeman, Eleanor
1994 "Perception of female body shapes as a function of exercise", in: *Journal of Social Behavior and Personality,* 9: 335-352.

Gergen, Kenneth
1991 *The saturated self: Dilemmas of identity in contemporary life,* Basic Books: New York.

Gold, Ron
1995 "Why we need to rethink AIDS education for gay men", in: *AIDS Care,* 7: 11-19.

Gu, Edward
1996 "The irrationalistic view of aesthetic freedom and the philosophical sources of social discontent of Liu Xiaobo."

Hamilton, Malcolm, Waddington, Peter, Gregory, Susan and Walker, Ann
1995 "Eat, drink and be saved: the spiritual significance of alternative diets", in: *Social Compass,* 42: 497-511.

Hartley, Pat
1996 "Does health education promote eating disorders?", in: *European Eating Disorders Review,* 4(1): 3-11.

Hughes, Peter
1996 "Last post. Alternatives to postmodernism", 182-188.

Johnson, Natalie, Boyle, Catherine and Heller, Richard
1995 "Leisure-time physical activity and other health behaviours: are they needed", in: *Australian Journal of Public Health,* 19: 69-75.

Kelly, Michael and Field, David
1996 "Medical sociology, chronic illness and the body", in: *Sociology of Health and Illness,* 18: 241-257.

Khushf, George
1996 "Post-modern refelections on the ethics of naming", in: J. L. Peset and D. Gracia (eds.): *The ethics of diagnosis,* Kluwer: New York.

Kirkwood, William and Brown, Dan
1995 "Public communication about the causes of disease: the rhetoric of responsibility", in: *Journal of Communication,* 45: 55-76.

Kirmayer, Lawrence
1994 "Symptom attribution in cultural perspective", in: *Canadian Journal of Psychiatry,* 39: 584-595.

Lewis, J. Lowell
1995 "Genre and embodiment: from Brazilian Capoeira to the ethnology of human movement", in: *Cultural Anthropology,* 10: 221-243.

Lynch, P.
1995 "Adolescent smoking – an alternative perspective using personal construct theory", in: *Health Education Research*, 10: 187-198.

Madigan, Ruth and Munro, Moira
1996 "'House beautiful': Style and consumption in the home", in: *Sociology,* 30: 41-57.

Martin, Emily
1996 "The society of flows and the flows of culture", in: *Critique of Anthropology*, 16(1): 49-56.

McRobbie, Angela
1996 "All the world's a stage, screen or magazine: when culture is the logic of late capitalism", in: *Media, Culture and Society,* 18: 335-342.

Meillier, L., Lund, A. and Kok, G.
1996 "Reactions to health education among men", in: *Health Education Research*, 11: 107-115.

Milburn, Kathryn
1996 "The importance of lay theorising for health promotion research and practice", in: *Health Promotion International,* 11: 41-46.

Montelpare, William and Kanters, Michael
1994 "Symptom reporting, perceived health and leisure pursuits", in: *Health Values,* 18: 34-40.

Nguyen, Minh, Otis, Joanne and Potvin, Louise
1996 "Determinants of intention to adopt a low-fat diet in men 30 to 60 years old: implications for health promotion", in: *American Journal of Health Promotion,* 10: 201-207.

Pinell, Patrice
1996 "Modern medicine and the civilising process", in: *Sociology of Health and Illness,* 18: 1-16.

Popay, Jennie and Williams, Gareth
1996 "Public health research and lay knowledge", in: *Social Science and Medicine*, 42(5): 759-768.

Radley, Alan and Billig, Michael
1996 "Accounts of health and illness: dilemmas and representations", in: *Sociology of Health and Illness,* 18: 220-240.

Rasmussen, Susan
1996 "Matters of taste: Food, eating, and reflections on 'The Body Politic' in Tuareg society", in: *Journal of Anthropological Research,* 52: 61-83.

Santiago-Irizarry, Vilma
1996 "Culture as cure", in: *Cultural Anthropology,* 11(1): 3-24.

Schwalbe, M.
1993 "Goffman against postmodernism: emotion and the reality of the self", in: *Symbolic Interaction,* 16: 333-350.

Spickard, James
1994 "Body, Nature and Culture in Spiritual Healing", in: H. Johannessen, S. Gosvig Olesen and J. Østergård Andersen (eds.): *Studies in Alternative Therapy 2. Body and Nature,* pp. 65-81, Odense University Press: Odense, Denmark.

Starrett, Gregory
1995 "The hexis of interpretation: Islam and the body in the Egyptian popular school", in: *American Ethnologist,* 22: 953-969.

Stokols, Daniel, Allen, Judd and Bellingham, Richard
1996 "The social ecology of health promotion: implications for research and practice", in: *American Journal of Health Promotion*, 10(4): 247-251.

Stravynski, Ariel and O'Connor, Kieren
1995 "Understanding and managing abnormal behavior: The need for a clinical science", in: *The Journal of Psychology,* 129: 605-620.

Tinsley, Howard and Eldredge, Barbara
1995 "Psychological benefits of leisure participation: a taxonomy of leisure activities based on their need-gratifying properties", in: *Journal of Counselling Psychology,* 42: 123-132.

Træen, Bente
1995 "Life style patterns among urban café guests in Norway", in: *Addiction Research,* 3: 123-134.

Tsouyopoulos, Nelly
1984 "German philosophy and the rise of modern clinical medicine", in: *Theoretical Medicine,* 5: 345-347.

Turner, Terence
1995 "Social body and embodied subject: bodiliness, subjectivity, and sociality among the Kayapo", in: *Cultural Anthropologist,* 10: 143-170.

Vågerö, Denny
1994 "Equity and efficiency in health reform. A European view", in: *Social Science and Medicine,* 39: 1203-1210.

van der Geest, S.
1994 "Christ as a pharmacist: medical symbols in German devotion", *Social Science and Medicine,* 39: 727-732.

Wallulis, Jerald
1994 "The complexity of bodily feeling", in: *Human Studies,* 37: 373-380.

Warde, Alan
1994 "Consumption, identity formation and uncertainty", in: *Sociology,* 28: 877-898.

Wenglert, Leif and Rosén, Anne-Sofie
1995 "Optimism, self-esteem, mood and subjective health", in: *Personal and Individual Difference,* 18: 653-661.

Medical Paradigms

Quality in Clinical Holistic Medicine – Criteria, Assessment and Handling

by Palle Gad

Quality in clinical medical performance is paramount. Medical science has been developed and elaborated during the 20th century and has captured a position based on tradition and acting as a monopoly on recognizing and administrating professional quality. At present, other reference criteria or qualities are not officially appreciated.

The apparent stringency and logic which we meet in traditional medicine derives from the quantifications, the dominating use of figures, which in turn facilitates statistical manoeuvres and neat in-one-glance-presentations: when authors or speakers have done their homework, the reader or listener can lean back, watch out for calculated significances, and so be taught what should be recognized as quality and applied during daily life activities. It is also a basic attitude that what is not paradigmatically acceptable is considered nonexisting.

Another typical trait of traditional sciences is a confidence in the objectivity of the scientist and his value neutral attitudes. Accordingly, the quality aspect has been connected to therapies, to the techniques applied, to the effects and to effectiveness. Individual evaluation of a producer of a certain therapy, on the other hand, has been informal and not exposed to the same level of interest; it has resulted in (single) cases of underqualified medical persons and also in late withdrawal of authorization in cases of gradually appearing incompetence or malpractice.

During the last few years, however, signs have appeared that the positivistic strongholds are relaxing (Almind 1996, Lunde 1993). The upcoming paradigm, the holistic approach to medical clinical activities, will use quantification where feasible, but will not limit itself to such a narrow concept. On the contrary, soft data (the everyday term for qualitative and nonnumeric data), are relevant and will be in operation to a much larger extent than hitherto.

One side of the discourse sketched above is the person aspect. The supporters of positivistic paradigms will only reluctantly recognize any other type of medical education; attempts to acknowledge qualifications of personality, especially, will be watched with circumspection, even disgust. Accordingly, we still meet orthodoxly educated people that prefer not to be seen in company with, and will under no circumstance cooperate with, non-authorized persons.

In the still dominating natural sciences, including medical science, the positivistic ideal is that the observer is bound to be and to behave as a neutral function, external to the observed object. The popularity of the controlled clinical trial may be understood from this perspective.

However, in biological, psychological and sociological matters all parts involved in a project influence the outcome. Even the observer of an experiment in classical physics cannot avoid being involved, a point of view brought out by leading physicists such as Niels Bohr (1885-1962). Therefore, in the future, it will be wise to include evaluation of personal characteristics of individuals in the quality criteria.

Furthermore, it is a fact that also holistic clinicians will be in trouble when deciding which 'colleagues' to rely on, because of the multiplicity and diversity of techniques, educations and philosophies available in an uncontrolled market of therapies.

Purpose of this Presentation

A meaningful step in the progress of holistic medicine is, therefore, the development of a set of acceptable operational criteria of quality and of practice in their application, with the purpose of examining and authorizing individuals as reliable holistic medical workers. This paper presents some experiences in an attempt to achieve such qualitative objectives.

Organisational Background

In the mid-1980s the Danish Society for Integrated Medicine (DSfIM) was formed, following generally accepted principles for medical societies around the world. A great number, but not all, medical societies enroll professionals only, i.e., traditionally educated and authorized individuals. DSfIM accepts nonprofessionals as members. The list of members accordingly contained a broad variety of interested persons, all types of authorized medical and paramedical persons, alternative therapists of all branches, and lay people, enthusiastic users, etc. Recently DSfIM ran into great troubles of various kinds, mostly economical and practical, however, none of them relevant to the present presentation.

Clinical experience and ambitions concerning the provision, maintenance and presentation to the public of a level of quality among therapists led to the establishment of a "Holistic Network". This substructure seems likely to survive the succumbing DSfIM, to be inherited by a new society to propagate the philosophies, etc., of holistic medicine. The organisational relation between DSfIM and Holistic Network was based on ordinary principles of democracy, i.e., the general assembly of the society elects an executive committee. The Executive Committee (EC) appoints three to five members of the Admissions Committee (AC); EC also supervises the overall activities concerning admissions, including the handling of possible complaints against decisions of the AC. Membership of the AC will not exceed 3-5 years, and running exchanges are possible. Care has been taken to have different professional branches, orthodox and non-orthodox, represented on the committee.

The criteria were laid down following preparation in a working party and a general debate in DSfIM. The philosophical background considered five fundamental aspects of therapies:

- medicine (including social medicine),
- biological therapies (i.e., nutrition and herbal medicine),
- structural therapies (i.e., chiropractic, massage),
- energy therapy (i.e., reflexology, healing, acupuncture),
- psychotherapies (i.e., gestalt- and dream work).

These five main trends of therapies are considered to follow the understanding of the five levels of human being. This combined philosophical and practical approach can be traced back several thousand years to Pantajali, one of the founders of the Indian yoga tradition (Petersen 1989).

This verbalization into a model of therapeutic everyday life is now being replaced by a model which intends to focus on patient's needs more than therapist's abilities. Such renewal is another symptom of the fact that this paper deals with a subject under development.

Thus, at present, the philosophical framing is suggested (Gad 1995) as:

The human individual, the HOLOS, may be considered as
- a SOMA entity (physics, chemistry, biochemistry),
- a PSYCHE entity,
- a ENERGOS entity,
- a SPIRIT, or a spiritual individuality.

These four aspects, each important in their own right, are inseparable in the concept of holistic medicine; whenever the focus is directed at, say energetic aspects of the patient's situation, the other three must be kept in mind. The distinction, however, is useful for practical purposes, and, for example, didactics.

Quality Criteria

Returning to the central issue of this presentation, the quality criteria, they can be formulated in five 'area headings'. The qualifications from all areas are to be evaluated as a whole.

A basic education
Preferably in the health area, but not necessarily so. The point is that the applicant has been able to complete an education at a certain level, through a certain length of time, having thereby passed a formal, final examination, leading to occupational competence in a traditional sense.

One or several side educations or trainings
The point here is that capability in a holistic sense can be achieved only through competence along more than a single track, orthodox or non-orthodox. The holistic therapist has to be familiar with more than one professional tongue, has to be acquainted with more than one therapeutic culture and their people. This will facilitate, when relevant in clinical practice, the referral of patients to colleagues of other specialities. Also, knowledge of possible accomplishments of other specialities will encourage sound, critical considerations of one's own major therapeutic direction.

Clinical experience
Only through the challenges of everyday work with patients/customers (which may be called 'confrontation') will one be able to learn what is common, what is difficult, even beyond one's reach, what will take time and what may be accomplished quickly. A general impression of life as a therapist cannot be taught at university, but only at the 'school of life' itself. Similarly, the handling of complications and unforeseen events is an important issue in achieving what we want to recognize in the qualified holistic therapist.[1]

---

[1] The principles mentioned under *basic education*, *side education* and *clinical experience* are very much the same as demanded from the Danish National Health Service to qualify for authorization in orthodox medical specialities.

Performance in general
This broad term covers a diversity of items, such as how the applicant presents him/herself towards the public (advertisements, brochures, for instance); the impression of personal appearance, including language and the use of language in conversation; price politics; standards in physical surroundings. And whatever else may be relevant.

Personal development
The holistic applicant will be able to demonstrate concern for and some activity aiming at his/her own continued progress, as a human and as a professional: holism means a never ending process.

The Procedure

The applicant will produce a written presentation elaborating on the five headings above. Then follows a personal appearance before the Admissions Committee. The conversation, concerned and still relaxed, which is supposed to allow a two-way exchange of information, will last about one hour. During that time the contents of the written application will be explored and supplemented, explained if necessary, and general as well as specific clues obtained.

Immediately after this conversation the committee members will seek consensus: accepted, accepted on conditions, or refused. The decision is referred by letter, which in case of 'not accepted' will include a short motivation, eventually including advice on how to improve possibilities for a later approval.

The costs of the administration and of the meeting (travel expenses, handling, etc.) will be covered by an applicants fee: a (symbolic) allowance to the committee members tends to strengthen professionalism during the procedure.

Experience

The activity of the Admissions Committee up till now shows that the efforts invested have been worthwhile. Two major obstacles for the applicants have appeared to lie in the (absent) training in psychotherapy and in the area of personal development.

From the skills of the psychotherapist one should obtain an ability to lead conversations in general to the benefit of any other participant; a quality which can hardly be overestimated, and which has not been taught at medical schools up till now, nor at non-orthodox schools.

In the area of 'personal development' the Admissions Committee will NOT act as a judge concerning what kind of activity is acceptable, but will make a note of any process and of the understanding of the applicant: does (s)he recognize the importance of the point?

As shown in this description we can account for qualifying 'positive' characteristics beforehand; a negative, disqualifying aspect, put forward by an aspirant is, on the contrary, not to prescribe. A disqualifying trait may be disclosed through the written application, but it is more likely to pop up during a personal interview. Therefore, the interview meeting with a three-person admissions committee is important.

Status

At present (early 1996) approximately 180 applicants have been accepted as members of Holistic Network. In about 15 cases, i.e., less than 10% of all applicants, the consensus resulted in a 'no thanks'; a similar number of applicants obtained a 'no thanks' plus advice on how to improve before a second attempt.

Members are encouraged to organize themselves in local basic groups with informal but regular meetings in order to get acquainted, exchange experiences, discuss their efforts in clinical daily life and in continued personal progress and to contribute to the life and functions of the national organization (DSfIM).

The nationwide membership list including therapeutic specialities of the members has a function in case of referral or information to the public.

Failures

Even if the Admissions Committee tries hard and seriously to keep high standards it must be foreseen that mistake(s) may occur, that an applicant is let in who later appears to be unacceptable.

It has occurred that a holistic networker did develop what seemed to be unacceptable behaviour and business politics: In both such cases the Executive Committee will ask the AC to summon the colleague for a renewed evaluation on the same basis as the initial application.

Complaints against the AC are to be foreseen, but have not yet appeared. In case of a complaint about a refusal, the AC is ready to state its reasons and is prepared to retire for a new set of members.

Discussion

During this retrospective study aimed at establishing criteria and their transformation into practical procedures, no report on any similar project has come to my attention. A literature search has not been performed.

However, during the writing of this report a discussion about the qualifications of Danish MDs in specialist practice is referred: A broadening of areas of skills is called for, but in the directions of business management and administration – nothing like training in psychotherapeutic conversation or personal development. The article appears to aim at more positivistic virtues, while holism is still avoided (Almind 1996: 320-321).

At the third INRAT Seminar (Copenhagen September 29th – October 1st, 1995) Vigdis Moe Christie (Oslo, Norway) reported some experiences from a 5-year effort of four orthodox and four non-orthodox medical therapists with monthly conversation meetings. The progress went from armed neutralism to mutual respect and cordial cooperation.

Establishing and maintaining quality criteria in professional performance is recognized as a delicate problem. This challenge seems to be met by the face to face meeting of aspirants and the Admissions Committee. Unforeseen combinations of qualities, positive and/or negative, can be detected and reacted upon.

National and local health authorities as well as the public are concerned, but will have to rely on professional advisors, which means colleagues of individuals. This will, in turn, always give rise to suspicion, doubts about whether and when to accept professional performance and evaluations of that performance. The free market forces will be in function, but this kind of regulating mechanism will in most cases not be satisfactory.

The described arrangement with a 'two layer' structure – the professionals of an admissions committee under supervision by the lay people of an executive committee (in turn referring to a general assembly) combines the peer review with democratic control and responsibility.

At first glance, the Danish governmental administration of authorization of medical specialists may appear similar to the Holistic Network approach. In two areas, however, the quality criteria of Holistic Network are more demanding than that of The National Health Service: Areas 4 and 5, general performance and continued personal development.

Besides the lay person control of a peer review, there is a third advantage: the procedure is cheap and even self-financing (as it is also self-administrating!).

In all the broad variety of branches of alternative medical therapies the same issues concerning quality are under debate. Different levels of professional and ethical evaluations have been set up, but none at the level of Holistic Network.

In this respect the obstacle most often seems to lie in the area of side education (area 2) and substantial clinical experience (area 3). The personal meeting is still unique.

In the area of law a parallel effort is making some headway, namely mediation: a practice aiming at resolving conflicts outside the courts, but with respect for human qualities; clearly this endeavour moves along the same lines as those of holistic medicine. In the USA some 20 years of experience in mediation has already been accumulated. Just recently initiatives have been taken to import the ideas and practice of mediation to Denmark (Boserup). An association has been founded (Dansk Forligsnævn), and it has been decided to follow a course parallel to that of Holistic Network in evaluating practising mediators.

Summary

A set of quality criteria to evaluate practising orthodox or non-orthodox performers of holistic medicine is described and compared with governmental procedure, especially concerning quality aspects.

Preliminary (approximately 5 years) experience is reported on. Lines of association are drawn with governmental practice on one side and alternative medicine on the other. A parallel effort in law practice, conflict solution by means of mediation, is mentioned.

References

Almind, Gert
1996 "Medicinsk forskning og klinisk praksis", in: *Ugeskrift for læger*, 158: 1989-90.

Boserup, Hans
1993 *Én konflikt, to vindere*, Dansk Forligsnævn.

Christie, Vigdis Moe
1996 "The Story of a Dialogue Group between Practitioners of Alternative (Traditional) and Modern (Western) Medicine in Norway", in: S. Gosvig Olesen & E. Høg (eds.): *Studies in Alternative Therapy 3. Communication in and about Alternative Therapies*, pp. 197-205, Odense University Press: Odense.

Gad, Palle
1995 "Sundhedssektoren", in: *New Age – kulturstrømning eller paradigmeskift?*, pp. 73-90, Munksgaard: Copenhagen.

Lunde, Inga Marie
1991 "Medicinsk-humanistisk forskning – genstandsfelt og metoder", in: *Ugeskrift for læger*, 154: 3-7.

Lunde, Inga Marie & Mainz, J.
1993 "Integrering af patientperspektiv i kvalitetsvurdering – en ny metode", in: *Nord. Med.*, 108: 121-3.

Petersen, Jens Erik Risom
1989 *Helhed bag dit helbred*, pp. 38-41, Borgen.

The Self-organization of Knowledge:
Paradigms of Knowledge and their Role in the Decision of what Counts as Legitimate Medical Practice

by Søren Brier

Abstract

This paper attempts to develop a non-reductionistic and transdisciplinary view on human knowing in the light of the growing development of interdisciplinary practices and sciences. Medicine is one of the oldest, ecology and information science are some of the newer examples on radical interdisciplinarity. In contrast to the classical mechanistic view of science, knowledge is in the new model seen as self-organized signification systems based on metaphysical frameworks communicated through signs with a meaning content based on social practice. The interpretation of a sign in a systematized knowledge framework is actually where the medical sciences started in the classical Greek tradition of Hippocrates. The paper discusses the lack of a recognized place and value of phenomenological knowledge in relation to the general mechanistic scientific ontology and its view of knowledge which is still central to mainstream Western medicine. The dualistic idea of transcendental and eternal mathematical natural laws and an algorithmic program behind intelligence and language is rejected for its lacking ability to include the phenomenological and existential perspective of knowledge and consciousness in the model, not to speak of the practical knowledge beyond words which is the level at which many so-called alternative medicine systems work. The new model promotes an epistemology which sees science as only one aspect of our knowledge, and sees human knowledge as going beyond language. An opening for the phenomenological is then created in our modern scientific and mechanistic metaphysics. This non-reductionistic framework promises to open towards a deeper understanding of the ideas behind many alternative paradigms of healing without giving up what we have gained through the rigor and the methods of the sciences and the logic of philosophical analysis.

Science and the Development of "World Formula Thinking"

Original semiotics, the understanding of how signs gain meaning through their interpretation as a part of a social-cultural practice, was a founding part of medicine. It is still in practice in diagnostication of patients' illnesses. But for hundreds of years medicine has built up its knowledge authority more and more on the classical mechanistic view of scientific knowledge, leaning most heavily on the chemical parts of biology such as biochemistry, genetics and physiology.

The idea of a purely objective (empirical-mathematical) knowledge appears to be inherent in the basic philosophy of modern science, as Galileo formulated it. By insisting that the exploration of the world is in itself good, that the major qualities in nature can be revealed by measurement, that mathematics is nature's language and finally that nature is basically composed of indivisible lumps of matter, atoms, the foundation was laid for an unhampered hunt for knowledge *in and behind* nature and for the conviction that true knowledge was not only revealed in books, but existed in nature itself.

In general, the kind of knowledge that has been produced through science and the development of technology during the last 400 years has become more and more central to the rationality of our culture as such. Christianity is leaving the central stronghold of being the true knowledge of our culture. Technological knowledge gives both power over nature and over others and is an intermediary between power and money. Science – and here especially natural science – has a double role in that it is both a technology developer and world-view producer. Faith in science as an instrument for obtaining knowledge of the world is an important part of the foundation of our faith in technology as the right means of developing society, and of "the modern world view". This is marked by an incoherent combination of empiricism and rationalism as epistemology and an ontology combining dualism with eliminative materialism in the form of physicalism imbedded in a theory of evolution believing in the 'self-organization' of matter.

A number of humanist researchers call this period we are leaving "the modern period". One of its characteristics is the faith in absolute objective knowledge as the highest value and the associated tendency to see science as a "great story". Empirical-mathematical science has, since Galileo, among others, formulated it in contrast to scholasticism's thought, become century after century an even greater part of our cultural self-understanding and world view. In that mechanistic world view lies a vision that Laplace formulated most clearly, about the possibility for achieving a complete mathematical description of the collective expression of "the Law of Nature": in short *a world formula* (Prigogine and Stengers 1986, Brier 1995a).

From my point of view, it is one of modern information society's main problems that there is an ideological tendency to view the acquisition of scientific knowledge as a unique and privileged path to truth and reality. All knowledge, other than "laws of nature" determined by physics and mathematics, is regarded as uncertain and subjective. A part of our cultural project is to carry out a final uncovering of all "the laws of nature", to find the ultimate safe basis for the construction of objective, true and provable knowledge. Stone by stone we will construct 'the Cathedral of Truth' and reach the final realization and control of our own and the surrounding nature. It is this project more than any other that separates us from and – according to our own self-understanding – raises us above all other cultures, including those from which the alternative paradigms of existence, life, body, health and medicine originally come.

This science and technology belief, where science becomes a "great story", has a lot in common with traditional societies' myths and dogma-based cultures. The myth defines among other things, what true knowledge, true values and real beauty are. Instead of becoming a real liberating knowledge, science is to a certain degree raising its limited viewpoint to a dogma called: "the scientific world view", which now through the "Big Bang" theory, the theory of a "genetic program" governing life, and through "cognitive science" and "artificial intelligence" promises of finding the algorithms behind language and intelligence, and implementing them in the computer, attempts to control our whole view of reality (Brier 1992b, 1993b and 1995a).

From the French Age of Enlightenment's Encyclopedists through Comte's positivism and the ramifications of the Vienna Circle's logical positivism, the idea of true knowledge has been interpreted in a more and more rationalistic and materialistic direction, until we today have ended with the split portrayed by C. P. Snow (1963) between "the two cultures", where modern humanities stand weakly in divided specialization and often highly refined aestheticism opposite financial power joined with the scientific-technological system. The humanities are having a difficult time finding a common basis on which to formulate their value assumptions, since they neither wish to turn ethics into religion nor science, and further do not dare define its view of human nature beyond our modern linguistic-material view of consciousness.

My point (Brier 1995a) is, therefore, that there is an ideological connection between the mechanical philosophy of nature, the material growth philosophy, and our existential problems, both as a culture and as individuals, which go deeply into mind, body, life, illness and death. Behind this is, again, a more complex set of connections to our historical understanding of ours as the most highly developed culture ever.

It is well known that for a number of years environmentalists and ecologists have questioned the possibility of continued material growth because of pollution and the tremendous imbalances in the world which the eternal hunt for resources creates. But moreover, the mechanical philosophy of nature's rationality is experiencing an even stronger undermining influence inside science itself through the so-called paradigm shift in the natural and exact sciences.

Here, the work of formulating the new quantum mechanics has proven important. The discussions about Heisenberg's interdeterminancy principle, the problem of measurement in quantum mechanics and Bohr's complementarity theory reveal some cognitive limitations which quantum mechanics sets for traditional science. In later years Ilya Prigogine (Prigogine and Stengers 1985) has especially pointed to the limitations to classical science which thermodynamics' discovery of irreversibility and "the arrow of time" in physics have set. Further, he has claimed that thermodynamics is a more fundamental science than mechanics. This has led to a renewed discussion about the relationship between entropy and information. Ultimately, concepts such as non-linearity, chaos and unpredictability are establishing themselves as fundamental in science. Science has in relation to it's own self-understanding ended in a series of situations of powerlessness (Brier 1993b), which should lead to a reconsideration of what the status of scientific knowledge actually is.

But in spite of there being a still growing number of theoretical scientists and researchers who have acknowledged limitations in the scientific form of knowledge, the Laplacian ideology of "the world formula" still influences the headings around a series of larger research projects:

First, the work with the united quantum field theoretical formulation of all natural forces' and particles' basic dynamics in the common mathematical description that today goes under the name, *"the super string theory"*.

Secondly, the efforts to find and manipulate "the fundamental laws of life" through the uncovering of *"the genetic program" or "the genetic algorithms"*. The human genom project (HUGO) is a part of this type of science and considered essential to mainstream Western medicine.

Thirdly, a similar idea lies behind finding "the laws or algorithms behind human intelligence", and transferring them to computers to create *"artificial intelligence"*. The project's more sophisticated continuation in *"cognitive science"* and certain forms of *"information science"* are attempting to find a common algorithmic denominator for all cognitive activity including language. This project is strongly connected to the whole program of neuroscience and the project of finding mechanical/physical explanations of consciousness and mental illness.

I am of the opinion that these projects, which beyond any doubt produce useful knowledge in some aspects, show that faith in the unlimited possibilities of science's rationality is still an important ideological factor in parts of our culture;

even though an ever increasing number of scientists and philosophers of science have acknowledged the limitations of mathematical-empirical models. The projects behind gene splicing, artificial intelligence and "cognitive science", I think, show how these research paradigms join together with a belief in technology's unlimited possibilities, as solver of mankind's problems. This is also a very important trend in mainstream Western medical science and the pharmaceutical industry's development and production of chemical "magical bullets". As Hoffmeyer shows in "The natural history of society" (1982), we are socially inclined to bring our problems to a technologically solvable form which can be sold on the free market, even though they may basically be of an existential, psychological or social character. He calls it *the technical fix*. This strategy has only limited usefulness. For instance in the case of antibiotics we see that infection is a part of a greater ecological and evolutionary dynamic system, which can only be beaten for a while with chemicals.

Knowledge of natural science has a very high authority in today's society, to a certain degree at the cost of other forms of knowledge. This is evident in the importance attached to this form of knowledge in medical science as opposed to social-psychological knowledge of coping with illness and the nurses' knowledge of nursing. Philosophy of science is here a good way to obtain a reflective relationship to the value of quantitative and natural scientific "facts", "laws" and "models" in relation, for example, to insight into social and psychological processes, including ethical and aesthetic opinions, when one makes a decision. I want to open for a broader view of knowledge that might pave the way for an understanding of other medical strategies than our own and thus increase our critical insight. My point is that we have to find a view of knowledge that makes it possible for us to combine the different kinds of knowledge pertaining to a specific situation or problem in a reflective and arguable manner.

The Copernican Turn in the Understanding of Scientific Knowledge

Rationality has by now not only eradicated most superstitions, but has also taken with it most of our faith in our own personal insight. We do not dare believe what we know. We are not capable of putting enough drive, feelings and creativity behind our insights into society's economic, political, health and ecological problems to make the needed improvements. One of the reasons for this is that it is very difficult in our scientific culture to find a place for personal knowledge and existential wisdom.

Today, we are drowning in "knowledge" of numberless subjects, produced by an ever increasing number of dissertations. This knowledge is getting still more difficult to fit consistently together in a common scheme of "the laws of nature", although the public in general is made to believe that it all fits together nicely. This in turn turns around too easily to become the view that nothing fits or can be trusted, for example when problem areas turn out to be more complex than expected, as in the question of what is healthy or not healthy to eat. This is even worse since it removes any belief in systematic and reflected publically communicated knowledge and the possibility for critical minds to come to a viable insight.

Still more knowledge is produced under increasingly varying conceptual and methodological premises; Thomas Kuhn (1970) speaks of various *paradigms of science*. This means that within science there can be different attitudes towards the nature of a subject area and the methods to get reliable and useful knowledge about it. An example is the different paradigms in psychotherapy which evaluate physiological, phenomenological and sociological data very differently in the pursuit of proper descriptions and cures for mental illnesses.

I would like, in the present context, to extend this concept to paradigms of knowledge, in order to include the systematized practices of meditation, health and medical practices of other cultures, such as Ayur Veda from India. Paradigms of knowledge imply the view that other kinds of systematized, reflected and publically communicated knowledge than what we normally call science exist. Most distant from science are the different religious systems. They harness existential knowledge of values, faith and interpersonal relations. In between are different kinds of systematized medical and health practices such as family therapy, psychotherapy, reflexology, yoga, meditation and different forms of spiritual practices. These often have long written traditions and theoretical discussions of why something works in practice. Less controversial is a lot of practical knowledge about the use of the body and mind in healing. Here, part of the knowledge is tacit. It is very difficult to express in a public systematized way. You need to have "the feeling of it". You need to have "talent", "human insight" and "skill". This kind of skillful knowledge is an important part of what it takes to be a good physician and/or therapist. Further, a lot of the knowledge collected and systematized in the arts or humanities seems to be of a different qualitative kind than the knowledge produced in the sciences. But this therapeutic and existential knowledge is produced in other cultures with other metaphysical frameworks of the body, mind and reality. To our confusion some of it works – for instance acupuncture – although the energies and their maps in the body were unknown to us and only partly coincide with something we know (endorphins). The discovery of the Chi energy (still not fully recognized) and the acupuncture points may have been phenomenological and further developed through experiments and practice. It seems to operate at a level that lies between our normal Western concepts of body and mind. This further accentuates our problem of the nature and limits of traditional scientific methods and the knowledge it produces.

The main purpose of this paper is, in a short form, to suggest that "the Copernican alternative" in the philosophy of science can contribute to a new framework of how to view the serious parts of 'alternative medicine'. That is to say, the movement from the belief, simply put, that natural science had the capacity and was in the process of uncovering nature's basic and universal laws and thereby finally would be able to explain mankind and its cognitive ability – to an understanding that the basic human ability to acquire knowledge is a prerequisite for knowledge. That is to say that knowledge begins from ordinary daily human knowledge (represented in everyday language concepts) and from there widens, is tested (logically and empirically) and refined. Instead of viewing scientific knowledge as approaching the goal of "final truth", scientific knowledge can be seen as an island of rationality continually developing against a vast encircling sea of ignorance or potential knowledge. We do not know in which direction we are going, only that the island (our knowledge) becomes still greater, more detailed and more practical for certain purposes. But we discover constantly, through praxis, that our knowledge is incomplete, among other things through the unexpected "side-effects" that a number of our actions have, but also through erroneous attempts in the use of it in new areas (Brier 1995a, 1995b).

It is true that the precondition for any language is the existence of something "outside" it, which it is about. But we are not in a position a priori to claim that reality is material and entirely determined by non-teleological laws. Galilean science has dominated us for over 300 years. It has shown us that reality has aspects amenable to exact mathematical analysis. This has been an enormously productive insight. Even mind has its "sluggish" sides, especially when reflected in a primitive nervous system that may partly be described in terms of functional laws. However, this does not mean that the content of all behavior and language can be transferred to computers, as some functionalists and cognitivists seem to believe. There is a "background problem" of individual and historical origin. In both physics and psychology (especially the latter) what can be described formally has its background in what is not thus describable: the hypercomplex phenomena, which besides the predictable, the regular, comprise among other things the spontaneous, unpredictable, intentional and individual historical (Brier 1993b).

It is not only the so-called "outside" world that persists in surprising us with its complexity and spontaneity. It is also our so-called "inner" world, the "subconscious" complexity and spontaneity behind our acting in the world, including our communication. Already Freud pointed out that we did not have absolute control over the impulses generating speech. Both Lacan and Luhmann point out that the conscious 'I' in the sentence "I said it" is only a part of the 'I' behind the production of the linguistic expression. This basic incompleteness in our knowledge of ourselves, the unknown reasons for our actions and our lack of absolute conscious control over speech, is at the same time the prerequisite for our ability to say something new and to cognize something new. To be aware of this will – so to speak – lead us to start in the middle instead of at the extreme, not start with either the subject or the object, but start with the process of knowing (Brier 1992b, 1993a).

Developing a Framework to understand the Relation between Science and other Types of Knowledge

It is important for the sciences and for interdisciplinary practical sciences, such as medicine, to realize that the process of human knowing, language and meaning is more basic and "before" any science. Bateson's (1973) suggestion that *information is a difference which makes a difference*, seems to me to be the best offer of a very general but fruitful definition of information and through that to knowledge which includes both objective and subjective aspects. But it has to be supplemented by a theory of the carrier of information: signs and the system to which the difference makes a difference: the interpreter (Brier 1992b). Information and meaning in their broadest understanding only arise from those self-organized – or in the words of Maturana and Varela (1987) – "autopoietic systems" we call living, which have a practical and historical relationship with a domain of living. Drawing on the works of Gadamar and Heidegger, Winograd and Flores (1987) underline that the meaning/information content of a sign is determined by social practice in an historical context, as opposed to the rationalist idea of objective information sitting "out there" arranged in bits, just waiting to be picked up. This is in accordance with the views promoted in the pragmatic semiotics of Peirce and the pragmatic language philosophy of Wittgenstein (1958). See Brier (1992b and 1996) for further explanation.

It is important to retain, and take the consequences of, the philosophical insight that the basis of science is the human ability to gain or create knowledge through its conscious being and its ability to make meaningful basic distinctions and signify through sign creation and communication. Human knowing is the fountainhead of all the different kinds of knowledge systems. All the different kinds of knowledge, such as scientific, phenomenological and practical knowledge, are specializations of basic human knowledge, based on the ability to make distinctions (with survival value) and communicate them through everyday language. Normally, we distinguish between our natural surroundings, our social surroundings and our own inner life of thoughts, feelings and wants.

These can be seen as three qualitatively different aspects of reality or different worlds. Nature has a reality which seems to exist rather independently of our social and mental activity. Society, as our product through cooperation and communication with others, is a human world created through human interpretations and practice. Finally, our own inner world of feelings, wants and conscious thought seems to spring, although dependent in many ways on nature and society, from a partly independent source, the nature of which science has great problems understanding within the prevalent world view. Further, we have no direct empirical access to other people's "inner world" of emotions, willings and cognitions. Let me sum this up in a graphic model. See Figure 1.

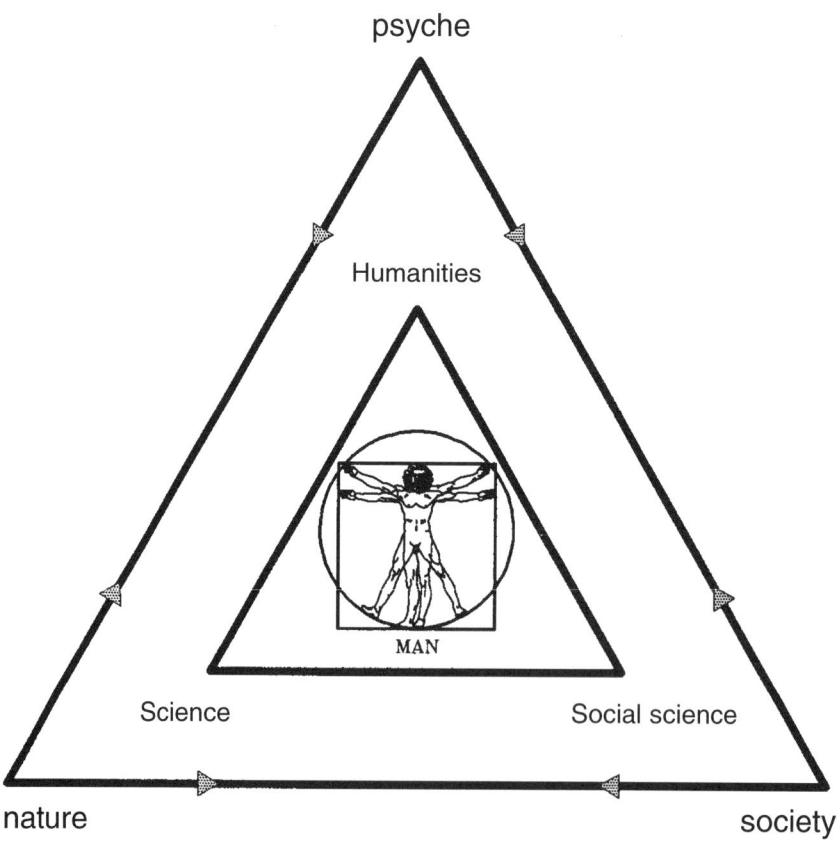

Figure 1: ***A graphic model of human knowing.***
*Reality is subdivided into: **Nature**, which is our material surroundings. **Society**, which is our human surroundings that basically present themselves in the field of language and rules of conduct. **Psyche**, which is our mind understood as our inner experience of our conscious thoughts, willings and feelings.*

In most cultures each of these subdivisions entails an authorized system of knowledge. The subject area and the interest of the research give rise to different kinds of knowledge systems:

> *Psyche:* to understand yourself: Hermeneutic-Phenomenological understanding: insight, qualitative self-knowledge: existential philosophy, psychology, systems of personal wisdom (mysticism and religions).
>
> *Society:* to understand the social relations: social sciences, anthropology, mythology.
>
> *Nature:* to understand the universe and its beings: natural sciences, cosmologies.

Now according to the mechanistic view of nature, mind and society there is one law, an algorithmic program behind it all, which science can find and produce on a computer. But according to Lindström (197?), as well as my own view and that of others, these different areas have basic qualitatively different ontological statuses and epistemological characters and therefore give rise to qualitatively different kinds of knowledge.

It is important to accept the unique quality of our inner world of emotions, perceptions, memories, theories and analogies, and that we at present cannot derive this world from either nature, society or a combination of them, although our inner worlds are clearly dependent on and formed by elements and processes from these worlds. As Lakoff (1989) shows so convincingly, our major way of ordering, understanding and predicting events is not logical or statistical but through motivated categories and connections.

Methodologically, we have no primary access to other people's inner worlds. We have only indirect access through physiological measures, behavioral descriptions and linguistic narrations reducing the complexity of our inner and outer world through meaning (making sense) (Brier 1993b, Brier 1995c, Luhmann 1990).

The social sciences have this double problem. They deal with interpreting individual persons but they want to find general laws for their behavior in groups. The attempt to found a genuine social science was an important drive behind Comte's formulation of positivism. Later, structuralism formulated by Levi Strauss and Noam Chomsky, among others, attempted to define an objective law-like social science. But Popper has in "The Poverty of Historism" argued at length for the impossibility of finding historical laws that can be used for predictions. His arguments are directed towards showing the uniqueness of historical events. He therefore also doubts that natural evolution can be considered a testable scientific theory as he defines it. The Dreyfus brothers (Dreyfus 1995) have – in the context of the discussion of the possibility of artificial intelligence – shown how dependent all social rules of behavior are on context (biological and social). Further, they have shown that context cannot be explicated sufficiently (for machine action) by laws. If you build several scenarios as different context, the machine still has to find out which one it is in when it has to interpret a sentence. To figure that out it needs another context on a higher level.

Wittgenstein (1958) has convincingly argued that the meaning of words and concepts depends on "language games" which are again a part of "life forms". Life forms are "things we do", developed praxis forms which can only be partly understood through "the language game of rule making".

So you have social sciences devoted to "case studies" of "the construction of meaning", for instance in therapy. You have refined mathematical macro-economic models built on the reduction called "economical man". You have Marxist and feminist research to reveal ideologies and power-structures with the goal of producing "emancipating knowledge". They all contribute to our understanding through different angles and qualities.

But there are other qualitatively different general systems of knowledge and expertise which intersect our general subdivisions of scientific knowledge. I have here used some basic terms from the philosophy of Aristotle which I will expand on below because many of our expressions have their roots there. It shows how old the problem is, and I think he has some good points in this division. To explain and understand this further I suggest – based on work in the "Danish Academy for Applied Philosophy" and Flyvbjerg[1] (1992) – that we reconsider Aristotle's three concepts of knowledge from "The Nicomacean Ethics" (Aristotle 1976): *Episteme*, *Techne* and *Phronesis*. In the English version, *Episteme* is translated as science (meaning the paradigm of classical mechanical natural science with its idea of eternal and reversible mathematical laws), *Techne* is translated as art (craftsmanship and 'know how' including aesthetic considerations) and *Phronesis* as prudence, understood as practical common sense (applied or practical philosophy including ethical considerations). Let us take a closer look at them.

---

1 Thanks to Bent Flyvbjerg and Ole Thyssen (Copenhagen School of Economics) for discussions on this subject. See Flyvbjerg's (1992) written discussion of the subject.

Aristotle writes about epistemic knowledge:

> "We all assume that what we know cannot be otherwise than it is, whereas in the case of things that may be otherwise, when they have passed out of view we can no longer tell whether they exist or not. Therefore the object of scientific knowledge is of necessity. Therefore it is eternal ... Induction introduces us to first principles and universals, while deduction starts from universals" (Aristotle 1976: 207 orign. 1139B18ff).

This is the ideal of science, coming from Socrates/Plato, further developed by Descartes and Kant during the Enlightenment, and in modern times by the young Wittgenstein and logical positivism. Scientific knowledge has to be: 1) explicit, 2) abstract (not depending on concrete examples), 3) universal, 4) discrete (composed of context-independent elements), 5) systematic (covering the whole subject area, connecting all the independent elements with laws), 6) able to make precise predictions. Modern medicine relies heavily on this idea of knowledge.

Techne, which is often translated as "art", is productive craftsmanship, construction of something, and relies on a blend of reasoned knowledge, know-how, tacit knowledge and aesthetic knowledge. Aristotle writes:

> "Every art is concerned with bringing something into being something that is capable either of being or of not being... For it is not with things that are to come to be of necessity that art is concerned nor with natural objects (because they have their origin in themselves)" (Aristotle 1976: 208).

You can imagine a spectrum with engineering at one pole and theater at the other. These are concrete, variable and context-dependent activities using practical rationality governed by a conscious goal of producing something artificial, useful and aesthetically pleasing (Flyvbjerg 1992: 72).

In contrast to this *phronesis*, often translated as prudence, is practical social and ethical knowledge used for instance in teaching, therapy, politics and leadership. It is pragmatic communicative social knowledge. Aristotle suggests we consider "a prudent man" to understand the nature of prudence (phronesis):

"..., it is thought to be the mark of a prudent man to be able to deliberate about things that are invariable. So... prudence cannot be science or art; not science because what can be done is variable..., and not art because action and production is generically different. For production aims at an end other than itself but this is impossible in the case of action, because the end is merely doing well. What remains, then, is that it is a true state, reasoned, and capable of action with regard to things that are good or bad for man" (Aristotle 1976: 209).

Phronesis then is applied or practical philosophy and one often thinks of leadership in state and private organizations. But it actually includes all kinds of social practices including medical practice such as communication skills in dealing with patients and how to treat a terminally ill person and her relatives. It demands deliberation, judgement and experience and it is context-dependent, related to the actual situation. Aristotle writes:

"Prudence is not concerned with universals only; it must also take cognizance of particulars, because it is concerned with conduct, and conduct has its sphere in particular circumstances. That is why some people who do not possess theoretical knowledge are more effective in action (especially if they are experienced) than others who do possess it" (Aristotle 1976: 213).

So *phronesis* has to do with social interactions between humans and is therefore an important part of any therapy carried out by people on other people. Some parts of medical practice are clearly *techne,* which brings forth something new and partly artificial, whether it is a new hip or a restored modern self-conscious ego. But we, of course, wish that these forms of practice rest as much as possible on the knowledge from science, social science and the humanities on which the best possible agreement is reached. See Figure 2 for the expanded knowledge model.

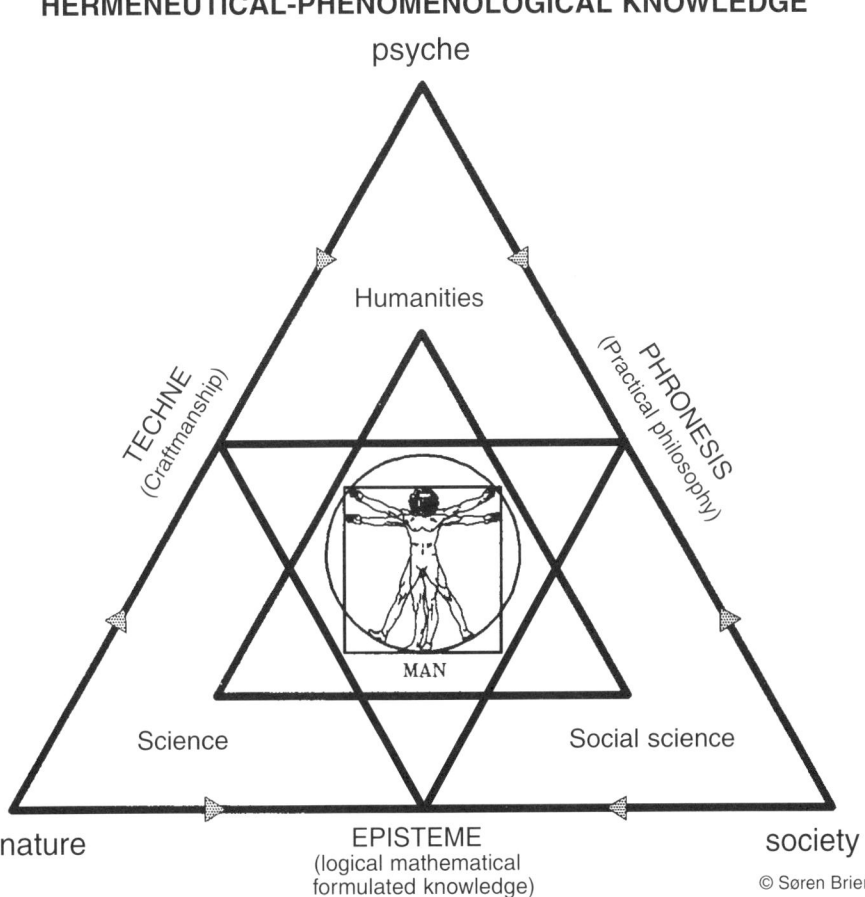

*Figure 2: **A graphic model of human knowing**.*
*In relation to figure 1 reality is now subdivided further into: **Episteme**, knowledge cast in logic and mathematics, which gives great manipulative power but is weak on contextuality and individuality. **Techne** is the ability to create things, art and health. **Phronesis** is the ability to manage well in social systems and situations such as therapy, teaching, communication and management.*

The model should – when also considering these three kinds of knowledge – be understood in the following way, taking epistemic knowledge as an example. It claims that certain aspects of nature and society are organized in such a way that epistemic knowledge gives us a fruitful representation of them, but that this is much less so with the psyche, especially the emotional and existential aspects of our "inner life" which are not easily represented in formal language. These are aspects of humanity which we have to describe in other kinds of language. The aspects of human nature most difficult to describe are those closest to the center. It is in the corners that we have developed languages for particular aspects of human reality.

By placing the human and its world in the center of the model, the figure also claims that we can only make models of human inner life, physiology, individual and social behavior. There does not seem to be support for the idea that all human action can be reduced to logical-mathematical laws. The fact that computer models are based on algorithms does not signify that nature, psyche or society as such is mathematical in its essence (see Searle 1985, Dreyfus and Dreyfus 1995 and Penrose 1996 for further discussion of this topic).

To place the human person in the center of the figure further illustrates what in cognitive science is called the idea of subsymbolic calculation (Hoffstader 1980), an idea now connected to neural networks, namely that knowledge springs from human beings as a cognitive individual before it is conscious rational symbol. Many cognitive activities are subsymbolic, that is to say, before any conscious formulation in symbols and language. The 'tacit knowledge' of Polanyi is one example, and Freud's idea of the unconscious is another example of non- or subsymbolic knowledge. Another way to distinguish this difference is between "declarative" and "procedural" knowledge, which is close to the difference between "knowing why" and "knowing how". The ideal of declarative knowledge is to describe the "Universe" in objective atomic and context free facts and the logical connections between them as for instance stated in the young Wittgenstein's "Tractatus Logico-Philosophicus". Originally, it is a view of knowledge developed by Plato and taken over in Aristotle's concept of *Episteme*. But "know-how" or *procedural knowledge* is connected to the human "world". Dreyfus et al (1995: 445) point to Heidegger's distinction between a "universe" and a "world" in the following quotation:

> "A set of interrelated facts may constitute a universe, like the physical universe, but it does not constitute a world. The latter, like the world of business, the world of theater, or the world of the physicist, is an organized body of objects, purposes, skills, and practices on the basis of which human activities have meaning or make sense. To see the difference one can contrast the meaningless physical universe with the meaningful world of the discipline of physics" (Dreyfus et al 1995: 435).

These different domains of human practice again only make sense against the background of a cultural common sense, which they presuppose. They are elaborations of the general common sense which they feed back into and thereby contribute to.

A Suggestion for a Transdisciplinary Framework for the Conception of Knowledge

The epistemic knowledge ideal – see Figure 1 – comes from the Pythagoreans, who thought that the whole numbers were the basic building blocks of the natural world. Plato used this ideal in his theory of ideas, where he considered mathematical ideas to be basic to the creation of the natural world (in the Timeios dialogue). Galilei used the idea of "mathematics as the language of nature" as one of the major philosophical foundations of the paradigm of natural science. The idea was developed further by Laplace and later Einstein and is seen in its extreme form in the super string project, the gene program idea, the vision of artificial intelligence and a cognitive science and in much current economic theorizing. The human being, nature and culture are attempted reduced to epistemic laws. This is what is normally called reductionism. It is important to notice, however, that reductionism is possible from all three corners of Figure 1. Whenever you claim that this is the only genuine kind of knowledge:

Study of psyche: subjective idealism, phenomenalism, solipsism.
Study of society: conventionalism, social constructivism, vulgar or mechanical historical materialism.
Study of nature: scientism, physicalism, materialism (mechanistic or dialectic).

The basic warning here is not to fall for any of them. They represent the temptation of the power of simplicity and fundamentalism. Our experience with both religious and scientific theories and paradigms is that they turn out to be fruitful for a certain subject area for some time and then as our experience expands new phenomena arise which the theory or paradigm cannot deal with in a consistent way. We then have to reconsider the philosophical foundation we started out on. We should not get too attached to either subject philosophy or social constructivism, behaviorism, cognitivism or biologism. They all have important knowledge but no final solutions. The problem areas' conceptual foundation and methods of getting knowledge, then, have to be rethought.

The late Danish philosopher of science, Johannes Witt-Hansen, stresses in his latest book (1980) the "situations of powerlessness" arising in science and the "postulates of impotence" they foster as crucial to the development of knowledge. He cites a number of examples in mathematics and physics. A classic example is the powerlessness of the Pythagoreans, faced with the realization that the side and the diagonal of a square are incommensurable, because it is impossible to measure the length of the diagonal of a square in units of the side, no matter how small these units are made. Today this relation is called the square root of two. The Pythagoreans were forced to give up the claim of their philosophy that the universe could be described as governed by harmonic relations between natural numbers. After a delay of two thousand years, this "powerlessness" was resolved by a fundamental extension of the concept of numbers to include irrational numbers.[2]

In physics, the realization of the impossibility of constructing a perpetual motion machine (perpetuum mobile) has had great importance to the development of thermodynamic concepts of energy and entropy.

In quantum mechanics, the recognition of our "powerlessness" to measure simultaneously a subatomic particle's position and momentum with an arbitrary precision led to Heisenberg's uncertainty relation and to Bohr's theory of complementarity.

With such examples, Witt-Hansen emphasizes the fact that situations rooted in powerlessness almost invariably lead to scientific revolution. Maybe the realization of the powerlessness of the mechanistic approach to psycho-somatic disease and the discovery of existential and psychological effects even on diseases long considered purely somatic, such as cancer, will provoke a new vision of the human body and the nature of disease.

Kant and Peirce (1892) have both insisted that science's "natural laws" do not exist totally independently of an observing subject. Karl Popper (1972) agrees with this. In his elaboration of Hume's arguments, Popper points out that no matter how many "repetitions" of an empirical phenomenon we have observed and predicted, we can never prove the existence of a universal natural law. This is because seeing "something repeat itself" is not objectively free of values, but is based on judgment of similarity. This judgment is always dependent on assumptions and interests. Repetition-for-us is based on a similarity-for-us experience. We can never demonstrate that the world of phenomena is inherently repetitious.

The consequence of scientific paradigm change in the 20th century is to a high degree scientists' acknowledgment that every work toward the construction of an exact model leads to the creation of non-knowledge or 'blindness' as Heidegger calls it. When we focus hard on one aspect of the world the others become blurred. They become "the background" or "noise". Every explication, clarification and formulation must always ignore aspects of reality. There will in this way, regardless of how much we exert ourselves, always exist objective scientific ignorance (Brier 1992b, 1995a, 1995b). This leads to a necessary opening towards other scientific and cognitive forms and includes an acknowledgment of the meaning of ethical and aesthetic considerations. But this does *not* give any

---

2 That is at least one way to narrate what happened.

real understanding of how these knowledge forms can play fruitfully together. Such an understanding will demand that we move up one level in the analysis.

On the one hand, we know that we have some knowledge, and that we can obtain more. On the other, we must admit that we do not have universal knowledge either in the physical sciences or in theology. Human knowledge is the meeting point between the subjective (individual) and the objective (universal), and so it is relational and prone to mistakes. It is an ongoing process.

We strive for universal knowledge. At least it is part of the ideal of theology and science. But the fact is that our knowledge is always contextual, and therefore limited to a part of reality. We are not even able to give a simple description of the limits of the truth-content in our knowledge (models, theories) in any absolute theoretical way before practical testing and attempts at falsification. To use a modern image: the border between the areas in which a given model makes true and untrue statements is not a smooth curve but seems rather to be a fractal one. So when we try to generalize knowledge it is always prone to failure. This is intrinsic to what we call human knowledge. If we could not know when we are mistaken, our knowledge could not grow. It is through our original ability to make distinctions in particular matters that we are able – by way of logic – to falsify our general models.

Science then seems to be our search for understandable and useful regularities and principles which organize and create natural things, including ourselves. This endeavor we pursue through the social construction of language, building on our fundamental gift of making (pre-scientific) distinctions in our world.

The Dane, Grue-Sørensen, in reflective analyses (Nordenboe 1977) pointed out the philosophical unsoundness of attempting to account for human consciousness in terms of physical determinism (which we have already dismissed). One cannot be a determinist because it is a true philosophy, but only because one is predestined by the physical chain of causes and effects. But in this way these views lose their logical and truth dimensions which are a prerequisite in the analysis of the views. Not only do they claim to be in accordance with the physical sciences, but they also claim to be logically valid and true. If one claims, on the other hand, based on thermodynamics and Bohr's measurement theory, that the universe is constructed by pure chance, then another kind of problem arises. One could ask how this world can exist at all and how scientific gathering of invariance is possible if the fundamental nature of reality is pure objective chance? If the world is totally governed by chance, how can any form of structure and law exist? Modern chaos theory and non-linearity is understood as a subtle interplay of chance and law, but that does not provide a solution to the fundamental problem of knowledge, reality and consciousness. Grue-Sørensen writes (Nordenboe 1977, note 61) about this problem:

> "The solution can only be found on a higher level, above determinism and indeterminism. One that does not contradict determinism in terms of the world of experience, but which turns it into a partial feature of a more extensive total point of view."

Peirce (1892b) – in opposition to most modern scientists, among them Prigogine – sees very clearly that the concept of chaos cannot be limited to the mechanistic concepts of a dead and mechanical world. You cannot remove in advance – so to speak – life and mind from the basic undifferentiated chaos from which worlds are initiated. Thus, he points out that *chaos is not the absence of law, it is the mother of law*. It is not empty, but full of possibilities. It is not only "dead"; it is also full of life and mind. Peirce coins a concept to explain at the same time evolution and regularities of nature. He writes that chaos has a tendency to be habit forming. Peirce therefore boldly calls it *pure spontaneity*! It is the spontaneity of living feeling. He writes:

> "On the other hand, by supposing the rigid exactitude of causation to yield, I care not how little – it be but a strictly infinitesimal amount – we gain room to insert mind into our scheme, and put it in the place where it is needed, into the position which, as the sole self-intelligible thing, it is entitled to occupy, that of the fountain of existence; and in so doing we resolve the problem of the connection of soul and body."

The final statement is perhaps a bit extravagant, but it is true that we long ago had to accept that a stimulus-response theory of learning within the framework of a mechanistic ontology would not aid us significantly in understanding what knowledge is and how it is at all possible. Since Descartes, the dualistic philosophy of mechanism has driven the spirit from the world and the world from the spirit and, as a result, encountered the most fearful problems in attempting to reunite them through knowledge. Peirce has another suggestion of ontology:

> "To undertake to account for anything by saying boldly that it is due to chance would, indeed, be futile. But this I do not do. I make use of chance chiefly to make room for a principle of generalization, or tendency to form habits, which I hold has produced all regularities. The mechanical philosopher leaves the whole specification of the world utterly unaccounted for, which is pretty nearly as bad as to boldly attribute it to chance. I attribute it altogether to chance, it is true, but to chance in the form of a spontaneity which is to some degree regular" (Peirce 1892a: 335-6).

Peirce (1891: 170) describes a possible model of the creation of order in the following way:

> "It would suppose that in the beginning, – infinitely remote, – there was a chaos of unpersonalized feeling, which being without connection or regularity would properly be without existence. This feeling, sporting here and there in pure arbitrariness, would have started the germ of a generalizing tendency. Its other sportings would be evanescent, but this would have a growing virtue. Thus, the tendency to habit would be started; and from this with the other principles of evolution all the regularities of the universe would be evolved. At any time, however, an element of pure chance survives and will remain ….".

In modern physical cosmology – the Big Bang theory and the super string theory – the universe is seen as arising from a random fluctuation in the vacuum field. It is very small in the beginning but rapidly it expands and thereby unfolds space-time. This is also the way in which modern quantum field physics describes the start of the development of the universe. The difference between Peirce's view and this is that most modern physicists believe that chaos is non-living and non-mental, where I, with Peirce, suggest a non-reductionist strategy by not starting by depriving reality of the living feeling, as Peirce calls it. In the modern view the phenomenon of life is intrinsically dependent on the basic features and dynamics of the universe.

In the Monist papers and other places (Buchler 1955), Peirce argues for a general triadic philosophy where *interpretants* create knowledge of different aspects of *objects* pointed out through *representamens* (or primary signs). The interpretant is another sign created in our mind through an ongoing process in our world and its connection to all the other human worlds that make up our cultural world. This unlimited semiosis is a never-ending process. The firstness of the representamen will first appear to us when we are concretely confronted with the difference in reality as they perpetuate our existence and make us interpret them to mediate or create a meaningful order (for us). For Peirce, logic and semiosis are attempts at coming to agree on a view of order or law throughout the whole culture. Logic is a social commitment. He points out that you cannot give a fruitful description of the production of signs and their meaning without a triadic basis (see for instance Buchler 1955). Thus, we do not deny the existence of something "outside" our *worlds*. Neither do we deny that it has regularities or habits so when viewed in certain ways it appears as a *universe*. But as there are many worlds of knowledge, we might better, with Maturana and Varela (1986), speak of a *Multiversa*.

General Conclusion for the Medical and Healing Sciences and Practices

Although it is a good thing to learn from the rigor in method and analytical rationality which has been developed in the sciences, the medical and health area in my opinion is basically interdisciplinary, including aspects both from the sciences, the humanities and the social sciences. It is well to keep in mind that a major point will be to attempt to integrate scientific thinking with social and psychological perspectives in both theory and practice. It is important to counteract the tendency to invest all authority in scientific knowledge within the medical area. I have made an attempt to formulate a new integrative but non-reductionistic perspective on human knowing, which includes creative and existential perspectives, *techne* and *phronesis*. In this age of artificial intelligence and the exponential growth of technology, it is important to restore authority to human knowledge and expertise. This does not mean that we should not conduct scientific research in medical problem areas. But it should be a much more humble project. It should, among other things, be the *social science* of how illness is produced, used, stored and constantly developed in the ever changing systems of a society and its historical and cultural contexts, and it should be the *phenomenological study of the psychological and existential aspects of bodyhood,* of relating the knowledge structure of the patient to the structures of the socio-cultural system in a way relating to the actual problem situation and the existential freedom of the individual.

The major problem in the medical and health sciences is therefore not to find "the laws of illness or health", but to cause theoretical knowledge from very different areas of research to interact with practical experience in a fruitful and practical way in relation to some goals defined in cooperation with the existentiality of the individual human person in the present unique situation. This can only be done well enough within a non-reductionistic framework for interdisciplinary work, and in interaction between theory and practice which is broad enough to make us conceptualize and understand other traditions of healing which may work inside the category which so far has been named 'placebo'.

I have suggested here a frame which is able to give context and meaning to a lot of "alternative" medical practices originating in other cultures, without being incompatible with the *results of science and the methods of science,* although it violates the common sense metaphysics of science. There is no way to prove that any metaphysics is true in the big sense. One must, of course, demand that it does not violate the knowledge we consider true and is in accordance with our practical experience. The other demand of this new expansion of our concepts is that it should include new areas of experience in a fruitful way that is compatible with our previous knowledge. The problems of including quantum phenomena in our scientific world view are no less difficult than accounting for the effects of certain alternative medical techniques, such as acupuncture. Both are changing our views of both the *universe* and the *world* and how they are connected.

Acknowledgments

Thanks to Axel Randrup (Center for Interdisciplinary Research, Svogerslev, Roskilde) and Søren Gosvig Olesen (The Royal Library of Denmark, Copenhagen) for constructive critique of an earlier version of this manuscript.

References

Aristotle
1976   "*The Nicomachean Ethics,* Penguin, Harmondsworth: London.

Bateson, G.
1973   *Steps to an Ecology of Mind,* Paladin: St. Albans, USA.
1980   *Mind and Nature,* Bantam Books.

Brier, S.
1992a   "A philosophy of science perspective – on the idea of a unifying information science" in: Vakkari, P. and B. Cronin (eds.): *Conceptions of library and information science: Historical, empirical and theoretical perspectives,* pp. 97-108, Taylor Graham.
1992b   "Information and Consciousness: A critique of the Mechanistic Foundation for the Concept of Information", in: *Cybernetics & Human Knowing,* 1(2/3): 71-94, Aalborg, Denmark.
1993a   "Conversational Ethics and the Global Environment", in: *Cybernetics & Human Knowing,* 1(4), Aalborg, Denmark.
1993b   "A Cybernetic and Semiotic View on a Galilean Theory of Psychology", in: *Cybernetics & Human Knowing,* 2(2): 31-45, Aalborg, Denmark.
1995a   *Verdensformlen der blev væk,* Aalborg Universitetsforlag: Ålborg, Denmark.
1995b   *Videnskabens Ø,* 3rd expanded edition, Nordisk Sommeruniversitet: Århus, Denmark.
1995c   "Cybersemiotics: On Autopoiesis, Code-duality and Sign Games in Bio-semiotics", in: *Cybernetics & Human Knowing,* 3(2): 3-14, Ålborg, Denmark.
1996   "Cybersemiotics: a new interdisciplinary development applied to the problems of knowledge organisation and document retrieval in information science", in: *Journal of Documentation,* 52(3): 296-344.

Buchler, J.
1955   *Philosophical Writings of Peirce: selected and edited with an introduction by Justus Buchler,* Dover Publications, Inc.: New York.

Christiansen, P. Voetmann
1995   *Habit Formation and the Thirdness of Signs,* IMFUFA. text no. 307, Roskilde University, Denmark.

Dreyfus, H. L. and Dreyfus, S. E.
1995 "Making a Mind vs. Modeling the Brain: AI Back at a Branchpoint", in: *Informatica*, 19: 425-444.

Flyvbjerg, B.
1992 *Rationalitet og Magt: Det konkretes Videnskab*, Bind 1, Akademisk Forlag: Denmark.

Hoffmeyer, J.
1982 *Samfundets Naturhistorie*, Rosinante: Charlottenlund, Denmark.
1993 *En snegl på vejen: Betydningens naturhistorie*, OmVerden/Rosinante: København.

Hoffstadter, D. R.
1983 "Artificial Intelligence: Subcognition as Computation" in: Machlup, F. and U. Mansfield (eds): *The Study of Information*, pp. 263-85, Wiley: New York.

Kirkeby, O. F.
1996 *Selvnødighedens filosofi*, Forlaget Modtryk.

Kuhn, T.
1970 "Scientific Revolutions", (Second Edition, Enlarged), The University of Chicago Press: Chicago and London.

Lakoff, G.
1987 *Women, Fire and Dangerous Things: What Categories Reveal about the Mind,* The University of Chicago Press: Chicago and London.

Lindström, J.
197? *Dialog och förståelse*, Avdelingen för Vetenskabsteori på Göteborg Universitet, Rapportserie.

Luhmann, N
1990 *Essays on Self-Reference*, Columbia University Press: New York.

Maturana, H. & Varela, F.
1986 *The Tree of Knowledge – The Biological Roots of Human Understanding*, Shambala Publishers: USA.

Monod, J.
1972 *Chance and Necessity*, Random Press.

Nordenboe, S. R.
1977 "Om forholdet mellem filosofi og pædagogik i Grue-Sørensens tænkning", in: Nordenboe, S. R. and A. F. Petersen (eds.): *Dansk Filosofi og Psykologi bind 2*, Filosofisk Institut, Københavns Universitet.

Peirce, C. S.
1891 "The Architecture of Theories", in: *The Monist*, 1(2).
1892a "The Doctrine of Necessity Examined", in: *The Monist*, April, 2(3): 321.
1892b "The Law of Mind", in: *The Monist*, July, 2(4): 553.
1893 "Evolutionary Love", in: *The Monist*, January, 3(2): 176.

Popper, K.
1972 *Objective Knowledge: An Evolutionary Approach*, At the Clarendon Press: Oxford.

Prigogine, I.
1980   *From Being to Becoming*, W. H. Freeman & Company: San Francisco.

Prigogine, I and Stengers, I.
1984   *Order out of Chaos*, Bantam Books: USA & Canada.

Searle, J.
1986   *Minds, Brains and Science*, Penguin Books.

Winograd, T. and Flores, F.
1987   *Understanding Computers and Cognition*, Ablex Publishing Corporation: Norwood, New Jersey.

Witt-Hansen, F.
1980   *Filosofi*, Gyldendal: København.

Wittgenstein, L.
1958   *Philosophical Investigation,* Third Edition, MacMillian Publishing Co. Inc.: New York.

The Connection between the Scope of Diagnosis and the User's Scope of Action
– Empirical Findings and Theoretical Perspectives

Laila Launsø

This article presents results of three research projects that deal with clients suffering from headache, allergy and cancer, respectively. The experience of clients with different treatments is set in perspective in terms of the concepts 'scope of diagnosis' and 'user's scope of action'. The scope of diagnosis relates to the context and the way in which the symptoms are understood. The user's scope of action relates to the person's perception of his/her ability and possibility to act in relation to the symptom(s). These concepts have to be understood as an abstraction based on users' experiences with different treatment systems. Both broad and narrow definitions of scope of diagnosis and scope of action are formulated and related to various knowledge systems. Consequences of different knowledge systems are described. Health policy implications are outlined as a conclusion to the article.

Users' Experiences with Different Treatments – Empirical Findings

Case
Jens is 28 years old. He is a white-collar employee in the marketing department of a major newspaper and works about 45 hours a week. He has a diagnosed migraine headache.

Jens started experiencing migraine headaches when he was about 15, and they have plagued him ever since. He had the worst attack when he was about 19. Jens' work is extremely demanding and he is convinced that it is vital for his body to function optimally. Jens used to take Treo (OTC pain reliever) and whatever else was on the market, but the pills did not help his migraine headaches. Jens says:

> "The last time I took pills on the job was four or five years ago, when I went around asking if anybody had anything for a headache. Then I took the pills and still had a headache and so what? … At some point you find

out that nothing happens anyway, so why should you take them? You just have to give up because it doesn't help. I haven't done anything about it. I don't like going to the doctor."

At some point, Jens decided that it was foolish not to try reflexology, because colleagues had told him that reflexology treatments can relieve headaches. Jens was treated seven times by a reflexologist, and his migraine headaches disappeared in the course of just over two months of treatment. At the start of treatment, Jens considered reflexology a kind of hocus-pocus. He was sceptical of results and did not think it would help him. Jens says he did all the things that usually trigger his migraine headaches in order to 'test' reflexology and see if the treatments worked. He went to bed late, stayed out a lot and drank plenty of coffee. However, he did not have a single migraine headache. He became convinced that reflexology can have an effect.

Case
Lone is 43 years old and carries a lot of responsibility in her job for a medium-size company. She has suffered from a diagnosed migraine and tension headaches for two years, with at least one attack weekly. In her experience, stress can trigger a headache. She has taken Panodil (OTC pain reliever), which has not brought any relief from pain.

When she was 12 years old, Lone was hospitalized for painful joints and treated with gold cure, tetracycline and prednisone. She has since been bothered by rheumatic pains in her back and legs, and she takes Salopyrine for the pain. Lone's doctor has told her that she will have to "learn to live with her headaches", and has in Lone's opinion been more interested in the rheumatism.

An occupational therapist at her workplace referred Lone to a reflexologist for her headaches. Lone had never had any alternative treatments before, but was willing to try. Lone found that the reflexology treatments relieved some of her rheumatic pain. After a treatment, she was able to sleep through the night, an unaccustomed pleasure that gave her more energy. She was able to reduce her intake of medicine. Her headaches stopped as well.

Results of a project[1] on headache, medication and reflexology treatments (Brendstrup & Launsø 1995a)
The two cases described above illustrate typical processes, as told by the clients. Most of the 220 clients we met in the project have taken headache medication

---

[1] 220 clients participated in the project and have been diagnosed by a physician consultant. The classification of the headache types of the clients is based on a headache diary and a registration form formulated on the basis of diagnostic criteria made by the International Society 1988 (Rasmussen 1994).

for several years in an attempt to relieve their migraine and/or tension headaches. The clients either experienced that the medication only took the edge off the pain or had no effect whatsoever. The scope of action known to clients in connection with their headaches was to try to forget them by taking medication. Headache has been perceived as an irritating, separate entity in the body. One client was told by a neurologist that her headaches were hereditary, and she was prescribed drugs as the most effective treatment available to her.

However, at some point, the headaches became too much for these clients. They decided that they had to do something different. They sought out reflexology treatment, often on the recommendation of colleagues or others. The fact that these clients wanted to drop headache medication and try other options cannot be seen in isolation from the demands their work and lifestyles place on their body-mind.

The effects of reflexology treatments develop differently for clients. What characterizes those clients who describe themselves as cured at the conclusion of the course of treatment, compared to those clients who describe themselves as not cured, is that they have been actively involved in the course of treatment. They have deliberated about what has happened to them during the course of treatment. Treatment has given them tools and insight into their bodies that they have been able to work with in the interests of prophylaxis. They have changed aspects of their daily life that they discovered to be inappropriate. Their former way of perceiving their headaches changed from having understood headache as a separate entity to understanding headache as part of the body and thus related to the body-mind and thus to their sociocultural context. In order for treatment to be considered effective by a client, the treatment must be tied to the person's concrete sociocultural context. The body-related effects of treatment must stand the test of ordinary daily life.

Results from a project on allergy (Hofmeister & Nielsen 1995)
This study focused on users of a biopath, a kinesiologist and a general practitioner (GP). The study indicates that those clients with allergy who had chosen alternative treatment exclusively at the time of the study felt that they lacked options for taking action within the established treatment system. Clients went to the biopath and the kinesiologist to gain knowledge and acquire tools that would allow them to act prophylactically on a daily basis. This scope of action derives from the expanded perception of allergy held by the biopath and the kinesiologist, which also incorporates the client as an agent.

It is noteworthy that those clients who choose biopathy or kinesiology as core treatment either become symptom-free or experience a dramatic reduction in symptoms, and they either stop taking medication or reduce the amount they take substantially.

Those clients who choose established treatments experience drug dependency, but the medication does indeed generally relieve their symptoms. Nonetheless, their attitude is critical, because either their symptoms have increased in strength and/or they are forced to continually increase their drug intake. Several clients have experienced noticeable adverse effects from medication. However, newer drugs seem to lead to fewer adverse effects.

Results from a cancer project at a centre for integrated medicine (Brendstrup & Launsø 1995 b)
For those clients we met at the centre for integrated medicine, the consequence of being diagnosed as having cancer and being prescribed surgery, chemotherapy or radiation was to begin considering what they themselves could do. These clients sought treatments outside the established treatment system in order to be able to do something themselves.

If we look at the reasons these clients give for the development of their cancers, we see focus on the breakdown of the immune system for various reasons. Some of the explanations given for immune system breakdown were: mononucleosis, genital warts, work stress, feeling inadequate, not being able to say "no", long-term use of malaria pills, unbalanced diet, large consumption of tinned meats, misuse of own resources, loss of loved one.

What clients expect from the centre is support in changing their diet and more information about what sort of diet can help rebuild the immune system. Finally, they expect 'a kick start' to help them change inappropriate living habits and to gain new opportunities to take an active part in and responsibility for treatment and the course of their illness. As practised at the centre, diagnosis allows room for the client's expectations. Those proposed treatments the client finds meaningful and effective are integrated into daily life, while the rest are dropped.

Clients perceive a healthy diet plus dietary supplements as one way of building up their immune system, as well as a way of counteracting the damage and adverse effects of established cancer treatments. Clients say that they do not think that their ways of living prior to coming to the centre were healthy enough. Diet is part of the daily scope of action for clients and they feel that they are making a concerted effort by changing their diet. However, a healthy diet is perceived as time-consuming to prepare, and obvious changes in diet or intake of dietary supplements are perceived as causing friends and family to react negatively.

In the course of treatment, clients experience that they gradually become better at taking care of themselves. They become better at decoding the signals of their bodies, at saying what they think and at setting limits in relation to work, social relationships and treatment proposals. Those clients who actively participate in and take responsibility for their own treatment evaluate themselves as being physically and psychologically stronger than when they started treatment.

At several consultations, practitioners spoke with clients about the importance of listening to their feelings and practising visualization at home. Most clients found themselves unable to carry out the latter suggestion, as they did not have sufficient experience with themselves on the psychological level. Positive psychological changes appeared along the way almost as side-benefits.

Clients were not ready to take full advantage of the scope of diagnosis offered by practitioners at the centre. Clients were focused on the somatic self as their point of access for taking action in relation to their cancer. In their experience, there was plenty to do on the physical level.

Theoretical Perspectives

The connection between scope of diagnosis and the user's scope of action
In the results of the studies described above, across the lines of client-experiences with various treatments, there is a connection between what I call the scope of diagnosis, and the user's scope of action. The narrower the construction of the scope of diagnosis, the narrower the client's scope of action.

What happens to the clients of reflexology treatment who describe themselves as cured at the conclusion of the course of treatment, is that they move beyond the boundary of their earlier perception of their headache by developing new knowledge and actions: they move from 'living with' to 'working with' their headache. One could also say that these clients have shifted from believing that they could control headache through medication to engaging in a dialogue with their headache, understood as an integral part of their body-mind. The clients see themselves as important agents during the course of their illness and cure. Characteristic of these clients is that together with the practitioner, they develop an understanding of why they have headaches and what factors can trigger as well as prevent them. The scope of diagnosis and the scope of action are as moving from narrow ones to broader ones.

Clients suffering from allergies who choose established treatments as their core treatment and alternative treatments as a supplement perceive allergy as an entity separate from themselves and perceive their scope of action as a narrow one. They look upon allergy primarily as something to be controlled and mastered by the drug treatment prescribed by skilled doctors.

The clients that did not want an established diagnosis of their allergy and who chose biopathy or kinesiology as their core treatment are characterized as being very active in regard to their allergy. They are experiencing a development in their scope of action. They see allergy as part of themselves and related to their way of living. They see themselves as the most competent person to verbalize and act in relation to their allergy. The practitioner is experienced as a catalyst who empowers the clients' ability to act in their daily context.

In the established treatment system, cancer patients primarily meet diagnoses targeted at the cellular level. It is assumed that treatments such as chemotherapy, radiation and surgery, which are independent of the subject, can cure or treat cancer. The basis is a narrow scope of diagnosis which offers the patient the option of believing in the doctor and putting his body in the doctor's hands. The alternative treatment area enters the client's sphere of perception as an option for being able to actively participate in rebuilding a poorly functioning immune system.

Clients indicated that they had an objective relationship to their bodies: they acted on the basis of having a body that 'needed to be put right' via diet, dietary supplements, etc. A subjective relationship to the body, on the other hand, would mean that clients acted on the basis of being a body in an integrating process. However, during the course of treatment, clients began to get in touch with repressed feelings and to feel better psychologically.

The body-related experiences and eventual empowering potential of clients, which can be made proactive through verbal and active work with the users' experiences, have lived in the shadow of medical science as well as mainstream medical sociology. The biomedical scope of diagnosis represents a social construction of the body that excludes individual experiences with the social and organic body. The social power that could be imagined as being within body-related experiences has not been verbalized or activated, either individually or collectively: on the contrary a de-verbalization has taken place (Launsø 1996). The body-related experiences have been defined as symptoms to be medicalized and removed rather than something from which we could learn, individually and collectively. The biomedical model implies a perception of the body in which the body is considered a recipient that acts reactively rather than a creator that acts proactively (Isaksen 1995).

While the experience of clients inside the established treatment system is that a narrow diagnostic scope is defined (and chosen), the clients who participated in the three projects described above – involving reflexology, biopathy, kinesiology and treatment at a centre for integrated medicine – found that they were 'offered' a much larger scope of diagnosis in which physical, psychological, social and spiritual dimensions were incorporated, thus holding the potential for a wider scope of action.

Several users were not ready to take advantage of the greater scope of action offered, and thus chose proposed treatments according to their degree of readiness and what their sociocultural context 'allowed'. Any dramatic departures from what was usually 'accepted' in daily life were met with opposition.

The scope of diagnosis and scope of action that users meet in different treatment areas can be seen as deriving from the perceptions of illness/health with which the practitioners work. Here we are dealing with social constructions in which people are caught. It is first when these social constructions are experienced in the flesh, so to speak, that individuals gain a more conscious relationship to what they think is reasonable and what resonates with their way of life, particularly personal identity and what shapes identity. By using the concept of social construction I want to underline that we are not dealing with illness/health understandings as some kind of "objective" truths uncovered by science. Rather we are dealing with illness/health understandings created by human beings in a field of power and knowledge interests. A vital aspect of the meeting between user and practitioner should be to clarify the perception of illness/health that the practitioner believes in and practices, so that the user can choose and reject practitioners, perceptions of illness and treatments. This, however, demands a self-confrontation from the practitioners.

It can be difficult for users to deal with the social constructions presented within the scope of various alternative practitioners, according to our experience from several studies (Launsø 1988; Brendstrup & Launsø 1994/1995; Hofmeister & Nielsen 1995).

Perception of illness, understood as a social construction, is not only the expression of an individual consciousness and treatment, but also of a collective, cultural consciousness and action that permeates the individual and vice versa. It is also important to see the social construction as embedded in a continuous deconstruction and new construction process. The way the body-mind is interpreted plays a decisive role in the ongoing creation of self-identity. The way a person creates his self-identity (which involves interpreting oneself) could be perceived as decisive for the initiation of healing processes.

Further, I should like to point out that the scope of diagnosis and scope of action can also incorporate a human-ecological scope of diagnosis and scope of action in relation to illness/health.

We might pause here for a moment for a slight digression on the subject of treatment methods/cultivation methods in agriculture. There are parallels between our way of treating the earth, including cultivating crops, and our way of treating human illness.

With the rise of ecological agriculture, which has enjoyed marked success since the mid-1980s, it has become even more obvious that a part of alternative treatment and integrated medicine have traits in common with eco-agriculture, while established treatments have more in common with the development of conventional agriculture, with its emphasis on chemical fertilizers, pesticides and specialization. In both the conventional treatment system and conventional agriculture, people are experiencing risk factors which they try to react against by choosing alternative treatments and ecological products.

Ecological agriculture and a part of alternative treatment represent a watershed in our perception of nature, the body and illness, as well as questioning the ruling compulsion to master nature, the body and the earth.

In interviews with users of established and alternative practitioners, it is notable that numerous people make a connection between cultivating the earth and treating the body, understood as seeing the consequences of chemical agriculture on the illness and health of plants and animals as having parallels with the chemical consequences of the health-care sector on the illness and health of people. Further, the intake of drugs by human beings has serious negative effects (directly and indirectly) on the environment. We are here confronted with short- and long-term risk factors. Clients also experience a connection between the ecological products they consume and the promotion of health. In this perspective the scope of diagnosis and the user's scope of action can be developed further.

Paradigms and Knowledge Systems

The scope of diagnosis and the scope of action "carry" paradigms and knowledge systems. The narrow scope of diagnosis and scope of action experienced by users could be looked upon as embedded in the mechanistic objectifying paradigm:

THE MECHANISTIC OBJECTIFYING PARADIGM	
SCIENTIFIC IDEAL	Empirical testing of disease theories of causal relations. The relationship between researcher/ therapist is a subject-object relationship.
SOCIAL CONSTRUCTION OF REALITY	Disease is perceived as the results of universal laws. Treatment is standardized and defined by experts
RESEARCH ETHICS	Knowledge of universal laws as the basis for external regulation of disease.

The broader scope of diagnosis and scope of action experienced by users could be looked upon as embedded in a subject-oriented practice paradigm:

THE SUBJECT-ORIENTED PRACTICE PARADIGM

PRACTICAL IDEAL — Learning and personal growth regarding user and therapist take place through interpretation of subject-related content of meaning, experiences and 'objective' societal relationships which the subject must be perceived as a product of, and as a creator of. The subject has the possibility to change conditions or relate to conditions in new ways.

A subject-subject relationship between user and therapist. The therapist functions as a facilitator for mobilizing self-healing processes.

CONSTRUCTION OF REALITY — Illness is perceived as a signal of imbalance and conflicts which have not been processed.

Healing is a matter of a person's internal work on body and mind. This requires the development of the person's consciousness and it demands autonomy.

The focus is oriented towards the unique, thinking, feeling, acting subject (the user) as the most important factor in healing, and is oriented towards 'objective' registrations of the user's imbalances.

The outcome of treatment depends on the user's readiness to use the therapies as tools in a developing process.

The treatment must vary from user to user and is related to the user's context of life.

PRACTICAL ETHICS — The healing process is a matter of empowering the user to overcome barriers which produce illness. In this process the user is expected to be self-dependent and to some extent supported/ encouraged by the therapist.

(Launsø 1994)

The mechanistic objectifying scientific paradigm and the subject-oriented practice paradigm can further be considered as "carriers" of different knowledge systems, which means that research and practice inside different paradigms produce different knowledge.

A distinction could be made between:

1) An objectivistic knowledge system in which the mechanistic objectifying paradigm is enlisted.

2) A hermeneutic and action-oriented knowledge system in which the subject-oriented paradigm is enlisted.

The different knowledge systems should be perceived as ideal-typical and serve mainly as analytical orientations. An objectivistic knowledge system is produced through a course of treatment in which an attempt is made to master or control the illness/symptoms without involving subjectivity. Objectivistic knowledge has been tied to an assumption that illness phenomena could be defined as objects, that is, objects that exist independently of human recognition. Certain research types and designs as well as types of practice and quality criteria have been developed to produce empirical findings within this knowledge system. The objectivistic knowledge system has detached dependency from subject and context. All individualized intentions and all meaning are neutralized and deep-frozen in an anonymous world (Nerheim 1995:16) to which anonymous statistics belong.

Modern diagnostic and treatment methods make clients anonymous. This happens because the treatment techniques developed are expected to work in a 'nonverbal' context in which attempts are made to eliminate the patient's body-related experiences. One could say that the logic behind the development of these treatment techniques and related concepts is "closed", because the conditions for applying the technology and the concepts are defined independently of experience and are thus immune to subject-carried and situation-oriented revisions or corrections (Nerheim 1995). The fact that verbal meaning is generated through the actions of the body is also ignored.

One meets the objectivistic knowledge system in the treatment system when the human body is turned into the object of abstract knowledge production. The client can acquire "knowledge" about his or her illness based on so-called "objective" measurements. The neurologist might say to the client: your migraine is hereditary and the only solution is drugs. Or the general practitioner might say to the client: your allergy is chemical/somatic and the only solution is drugs. The oncologist might say to the client: your cancer must be treated at cell level and therefore I have to use chemotherapy and radiation. These statements represent a narrow scope of diagnosis, and one consequence may be that the client is left feeling paralysed (Brendstrup & Launsø 1995; Hofmeister & Nielsen 1995).

With its one-sided emphasis on objectivistic knowledge production, the treatment system has developed treatment technologies that have neither demanded nor allowed the client to be an agent involved in his own course of illness and healing. As a result, many users feel that they have lost their sovereignty over their body-mind, illness and healing. They find it difficult to take responsibility. In this connection, it gives food for thought that people who seek alternative treatment say that they want to have the chance to take responsibility for their body-mind, illness and health in the course of treatment they undergo (Launsø 1988, 1995; Brendstrup & Launsø 1993, 1994/95; Hofmeister & Nielsen 1995).

A hermeneutic and action-oriented knowledge system is produced through a course of treatment oriented towards providing scope for subjectivity (and the Self) through concepts such as self-realization, self-interpretation, self-reflection, self-expression and self-determination. Here, the understanding and experience of the body are given scope. Hermeneutic understanding involves changing or further developing one's horizon of understanding (Nerheim 1995: 281). Researching and treating illness require access with scope for subjective factors and external factors which can capture the subject's perspective on the world in which he or she lives. Here, the knowledge of the body is in primary focus. Headache, allergy or cancer is diagnosed in a scope that allows the potential for taking action, the scope for incorporating the client actively. This can be liberating for some clients and overwhelming for others (Hofmeister & Nielsen 1995; Brendstrup & Launsø 1995). Many people are shocked by how much is demanded of them, and many feel that they lack the requisite language and knowledge, which must thus be allowed time to develop (Launsø 1988; Brendstrup & Launsø 1994/95).

A hermeneutic and action-oriented knowledge system can be developed in a course of treatment in which people consciously process and integrate the body-mind in an exchange and development with their surroundings. The practices developed by practitioners are thus shaping people's bodies with consequences for developing their self-identity. In a manner of speaking, the body is at stake, as counter images to the image of the body in the established treatment system are generated when people encounter the above mentioned treatments: biopathy, kinesiology, reflexology and integrated medicine (Hofmeister & Nielsen 1995; Launsø et al (eds.) 1995; Brendstrup & Launsø 1995). In turn, this creates the platform for being able to develop a mode of resistance against the exercise of power many users encounter today in their meeting with the established treatment system.

Consequences of different knowledge systems
The two knowledge systems are based on different forms of rationalities. While the objectivistic knowledge system is based on technical rationality or mastery rationality, the hermeneutic and action-oriented knowledge system is based on communicative and pragmatic rationality, which deals with people's 'meeting' with themselves and their environments while working with both the meaning-carried symbols of language and action-oriented practice.

The object of treatment based on hermeneutic and action-oriented knowledge is to produce a conceptually pragmatic understanding dependent on subject and its sociocultural context, and it can lead to new insight and new ways of acting with an emancipating goal. A pragmatic understanding is related to whether treatment works and how it works for the individual in his/her sociocultural context.

The concept of effect is related to daily life and oriented towards learning and change with regard to the integration of physical, psychological, spiritual and social processes. Treatment can be recognized by its production of indirect and relational effects. The process of healing will be individual and it can be difficult and drawn out.

Naturally, one question that can be raised is whether the conditions for healing processes must be found within a hermeneutic and action-oriented knowledge system. Inherent in the system is the potential for developing a dialogue between user and practitioner. The crucial element in a hermeneutic dialogue is the creation of an 'intimate context' (Nerheim 1995) in which the results are not dictated by the practitioner.

At any rate, it is thought-provoking that knowledge of the processes of healing is nonexistent within an objectivistic knowledge system. At the same time, we must acknowledge that this knowledge system is important and powerful in our society today in regard to perception of illness and perception of treatment, and thus in relation to the definition of scope of diagnosis and the user's scope of action.

Another question that could be raised is whether the objectivistic knowledge system has tipped the balance between expert control and democratic control of the established treatment system (Wadskjær 1995). Many users seek alternative treatments that allow scope for democratic control. Many users want to be in charge and to have the scope to be the expert in terms of their own body-related experiences, preferences, requirements and goals for treatment. Therefore, many users want individual treatments that can be incorporated into their daily lives and values and contribute to the development of their personal identities. The present standard treatments are being increasingly challenged by these demands and others like them in future. At the societal level this challenge could be related to the theory of reflexive modernization (Beck 1995).

Health policy implications
The research referred to in the article identifies several priorities that need to be reordered in the health-care system:

1. Greater priority should be given to a scope of diagnosis and thus perceptions of illness that give users a greater scope of action. Conversely, lower priority should be given to narrow scopes of diagnosis and action.

2. Greater priority should be given to ecological and individual treatments of illness, in which the body-mind cannot be separated. Conversely, lower priority should be given to chemical and standardized techniques for combating illness. It will be necessary to study the scope of validity for the two types of treatment access, and their actual and potential risk factors.

3. Greater priority should be given to treatments that consider the connections between earth-nutrition-body-illness-health-society.

References

Beck, U.
1995 "The Reinvention of Politics: Towards a Theory of Reflexive Modernization", in: U. Beck, et al (eds.): *Reflexive Modernization. Politics, Traditions and Aesthetics in the Modern Social Order*, Polity Press: Cambridge.

Brendstrup, E. and Launsø, L.
1993 "Evaluation of a Non-drug Intervention Programme for Younger Seniors", in: *Journal of Social and Administrative Pharmacy*, 10(1): 23-35.
1994/5 "A Description of a Holistic Treatment Model – Used by Cancer Patients and Research Evaluated", in: *Townsend Letter for Doctors*, USA. Dec. 1994: 1342-56, Jan. 1995: 54-61.
1995a *Hovedpine og zoneterapeutisk behandling (Headache and reflexology treatment)*, The National Board of Health Council on Alternative Treatment. The National Board of Health, Copenhagen. (Is planned to be published in English 1997).
1995b "An Unconventional Cancer Treatment Model – a research project", (submitted 1996).

Isaksen, L. W.
1995   "Den sociale kroppen", in: Kjønn og samfunn i endring, [The social body. In: Gender and Society in Change]. Report from concluding conference, Norges Forskningsråd: Oslo.

Hofmeister, E., Launsø, L. and Brendstrup, E.
1994   *Centre for integreret medicin – alternativ behandling i udvikling* [Centres for Integrated Medicine – Alternative Treatment under Development], Department of Social Pharmacy, The Royal Danish School of Pharmacy: Copenhagen. (A summary is published in: Studies in Alternative Therapy – 1. Contributions from the Nordic Countries. Johannessen, Launsø, Olesen & Staugaard (ed.) Odense University Press, Odense, 1994.)

Hofmeister, E. and Nielsen, J. J.
1995   *Allergibehandlinger hos biopat, kinesiolog og alment praktiserende læge* [Allergy treatments by biopat, kinesiologist and general practitioner], The National Board of Health Council on Alternative Treatment, The National Board of Health: Copenhagen.

Launsø, L.
1988   *På vej mod integreret medicin – brugere og behandlere på Birkeholm*, [Towards integrated medicine – users and practitioners at Birkeholm, Center for Integrated Medicine], Aksigraf: Copenhagen.
1994   "How to kiss a monster! Design and Paradigmes in Research on Alternative Therapy", in: H. Johannessen, L. Launsø, S. Gosvig Olesen and F. Staugaard (eds.): *Studies in Alternative Therapy – 1. Contributions from the Nordic Countries*, Odense University Press: Odense.
1996   *Det alternative behandlingsområde. Brug og udvikling; rationalitet og paradigmer*, [The alternative treatment area. Use and development; rationality and paradigms], Akademisk Forlag: Copenhagen.

Launsø, L., Hofmeister E. and Bredstrup, E.
1995   "Centre for integreret medicin", in: L. Launsø, A. Tingstad and K. Skjerbæk, (eds.): *Livskraft og mennesker*, [Vitality and human beings], Akademisk Forlag: Copenhagen.

Nerheim, H.
1995   *Vitenskap og kommunikasjon. Paradigmer, modeller og kommunikative strategier i helsefagenes videnskabsteori*, [Science and communication. Paradigms, models and communication strategies in the scientific theories of the health care professions], Universitetsforlaget: Oslo.

Rasmussen, B.K.
1994   *Epidemiology of Headache*, University of Copenhagen: Copenhagen.

Wadskjœr, H.
1995   "Det moderne menneske – som borger og bruger", [The modern individual – as citizen and user], in: *Mit Helbred*, 35: 8-14.

Organic Agriculture and Alternative Medicine: Parallels and Paradigms

by Ane Bodil Søgaard

An increasing number of consumers are insecure and unsatisfied with the conventional foodstuffs and prefer ecologically produced goods. The fear of toxic and other foreign substances in food is widespread and well-founded. Physicians are quietly going over to prescribing unsprayed produce for the growing number of patients who suffer from arthritis and allergy. Ever more people augment their daily fare with minerals and other forms of diet supplements from health food stores. The alternative medical system is contacted by every third Dane.

Within the last forty to fifty years there has occurred such an emphatic increase in allergy, cancer and arthritis cases that, if the trend continues, in a very few years it will be more normal to be allergic than not. More and more people have problems of childlessness, and the sperm quality is dropping. The number of mentally ill in Denmark has doubled since 1950, with a consequent increase in the use of psychopharmaceuticals of which the Prozac-type happy pill is hopefully the culmination.

Within livestock production there are increasing difficulties with diseases, stress, quality, infertility, behavioral problems, cannibalism and at times signs of severe mental disorders. Particularly great are the problems within industrialized pig and poultry production, in which hormones, antibiotics and growth promoters in porker production and salmonella in chickens and eggs are among the front runners.

In Denmark the agricultural use of nitrogen just in the form of fertilizers has sextupled since 1950, and both the yield and the consumption of pesticides have risen at the same rate.

Reports of finds of nitrate and pesticides in the ground water are everyday reading in the newspapers, just as the dwindling ozone layer and the increasing CO_2 content in the atmosphere are current problems in connection with the global environment.

The past one-half to one year has seen the publication of voluminous reports and books on foodstuff quality, environment and health, both from the political as well as the scientific world (Landbrugs- og Fiskeriministeriet 1995, Land-

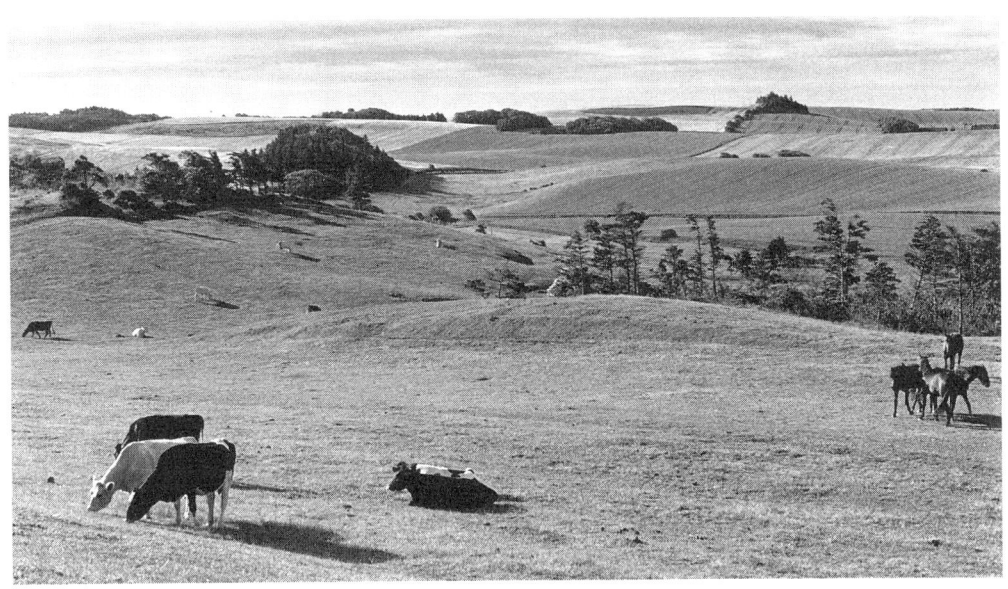

brugsrådet 1995, Miljø- og Energiministeriet 1995, Specialarbejderforbundet 1995). Most recently the Animal Ethics Council published a twenty-page critical pronouncement in November 1995, including a long series of proposed changes and restraints in connection with cattle, pig and poultry production.

A thought which immediately suggests itself is that there is a connection between the problems of disease, foodstuff quality, behavior, fertility, and air, soil and water pollution, as all of these problems have developed parallelly in time. It is merely that the connections are not so simple and direct that you can point at the one problem as cause and the other as effect. Perhaps it is rather that the problems are linked in the sense that they have the same cause in common.

Holistic scientific thinking began understandably enough within medicine, as the limits of reductionistic scientific thinking naturally are easiest to register where the consequences can be felt directly on one's own body.

Agronomics, more indirectly than medicine, has an influence on us and so it is no wonder that holistic thinking makes it appearance within agriculture, though somewhat delayed as compared to alternative medicine.

In the following I will illustrate with examples how the Western world's growth philosophy has had an influence on and affected conventional agriculture, its methods and view of the soil, plants, animals, quality and health. I will examine differences in conventional and ecological farming, and leave it to the reader to draw parallels to conventional and holistic medicine.

Growth and Madness

In conventional farming and market gardening the prevailing philosophy has been: as great a yield as possible. This view has legitimized a long series of expedients. More fertilizer gives a bigger yield. Therefore, as mentioned previously, the consumption of nitrogen, merely in the form of fertilizers, has sextupled per hectar farmland since 1950. Insect attacks and fungus diseases reduce the yield. So you counteract them by spraying. Weeds compete with the crop for light, water and nourishment, and therefore you spray them away with diverse chemical remedies.

The resulting effects are incalculable. To date there have been found in Denmark eight (Andreassen & Jensen 1994) and globally one hundred and twelve herbicide resistant species of weeds (Holt et al 1993). More and more ground water borings show nitrate and pesticide pollution. Among married couples where the man participates actively in spraying, there is a demonstrable connection between the spraying season and low reproductive ability (de Cock et al 1994). The incidence of skin and lung cancer is significantly higher among greenhouse gardeners compared with the rest of the population.

With copious application of nitrogen, nitrate is accumulated in the plants. Nitrate in itself is presumably non-toxic, but it is transformed into nitrite which is problematic. Even more unpleasant, in animal and human organisms nitrite can be transformed into nitrous amines, which are known for their carcinogenic properties.

Nearly all nutrients such as protein, fiber, most vitamins and minerals are diminished by the increased addition of nitrogen (Levnedsmiddelstyrelsen 1990). However, as mentioned the nitrite content is augmented in keeping with the increased supply of nitrogen, as is, most importantly, the yield. By way of example, the yield of wheat has increased from 4 to 7.5 t/ha, while barley has increased from a little more than 3 to 5.5 t/ha since 1950.

In addition to the nutrients most flavors, odors and aromas are also diminished by intensive cultivation (Toldam-Andersen & Hansen 1995). So by now it is a rarity to eat a tomato which tastes like tomato, and a cucumber which tastes like cucumber.

But most importantly – at any rate from a plant point of view – in keeping with the increasing supply of nitrogen many of the secondary substances that actively participate in plants' natural defence mechanisms against both fungi, insects and other herbivores, including ourselves, are reduced (Margna et al 1989). Thereby, the need increases – also for that reason – for employing plant protection agents.

Livestock farming has naturally been subject to the same basic assumption: the more growth the better. An average cow in 1950 gave ca. 10 litres of milk a day, while nowadays it gives at least the double. The connection between high milk yield and inflammation of the udder is one among the many costs of high milk production (Pounden & Frank 1961). It is "met" with antibiotics. Among other costs can be mentioned, for example, that a cow which yields 10 l milk per day has an 80% chance of becoming pregnant at the first insemination, whereas a cow which yields 20 l only has a 37% chance (Braun et al 1983).

In swine production one can see in retrospect that the first problems made their appearance around 1950. The phenomenon of the by now well-known very pale and watery meat was called muscle degeneration. However, this assumption was abandoned in favor of inherited susceptibility to "stress." Up through the fifties and sixties the number of stress sensitive animals rose – while at the same time the individual animal's stress sensitivity constantly increased. It took less and less stress to give rise to the pale and watery meat. Parallel with the increasing stress sensitivity, other problems turned up. Particularly, respiratory ailments with a chronic course took on disquieting dimensions, with increased medicine consumption as a result (Hansen & Hansen 1978).

Gradually, as all pigs went over to living exclusively from industrially manufactured feed, gastric ulcers and dysentary-like enteritis were also seen on a disquieting scale. Circulatory and cardiac failure increasingly became the cause of death of pigs.

In keeping with the increasingly more widespread "stress" sensitivity, fertility dropped off, requiring the use of hormone treatments. At the same time more and more serious behavioral disturbances were seen, which in their mildest form were displayed in abnormal nervousness, aggressiveness and tail biting. In the more extreme form, the pigs simply ate each other.

In the late sixties a new abnormality turned up in which the meat was dark, sticky and dry. At first this abnormality showed up only in the cold months, but in the course of the seventies the dark pork appeared at all seasons of the year and in increasingly large amounts. This dark quality of the meat was known from dead sick or destroyed animals, or animals butchered in a state of great exhaustion. The dark pork keeps badly because of an entire or partial absence of lactic acid, which reduces the meat's resistance to bacteria.

In order to reduce the steadily increasing medication costs, for example, a new stall system, SPF (specific patogene free), was introduced which could prevent or diminish the burden of contagion. In this production form, pigs live in isolation and are fed automatically. Since 1950, when a pig was supposed to grow ca. 600 g per day and until today when a corresponding pig must gain ca. 1 kg daily, pig problems are far from being solved. The addition of antibiotics to the feed has been augmented under the designation "growth promoter", with constantly more finds of resistant bacteria as a result. At the same time "natural" bacteria are now being added to industrial feed. It is hoped this will restore the original flavor to pork, after all the bacteria which occur naturally in a pig have been removed with antibiotics.

Nutrients

Plants have relatively simple requirements as to nourishment, inasmuch as they are able on the basis of water, light and a few substances to produce all of the amino acids, proteins, carbohydrates, fats, vitamins, minerals, hormones, odors and pigments, plus all of the other substances plants after all contain.

Both humans and livestock have a far greater complexity than plants. Even though there can also be differences in apples, for example, which come from the same tree and carrots which grow side by side, those differences, both with respect to nutrition and health, are far more intelligible than is the case among livestock, not to mention human beings.

Even in primitive agricultural societies it was known that by the addition of plant and animal remains, yield would be increased. As early as 1699 Woodward observed that plants survived and grew better in dirty water than in rainwater (Woodward 1699: 382).

Within plant physiology, in the early 1800s there were beginning investigations as to what substances plants had need of by cultivating them in water to which various substances had been added. And by mid-century the state of the knowledge was such that it had become clear that there were ten substances that were essential for plants: carbon, oxygen, hydrogen, nitrogen, phosphorus, potassium, calcium, sulphur, magnesium and iron.

Not until 1905 did Bertrand discover that manganese was also necessary for normal plant growth (Bertrand 1905). The next four substances boron, zink, copper and molybdenum did not become "necessary" for plants until just before the Second World War. Things did not stop there. We now know that at any rate some plants need sodium, aluminum, silicium, chlorine, gallium and cobolt, and experiments with legumes have revealed a need for chromium and nickle.

Many might wonder why even in the first hydroponic experiments it was not discovered that plants did not grow normally and therefore had to lack certain nutrients.

This is easier said than done. For example, how do you determine whether a plant has optimum conditions? That it has the best possible conditions for growth? How can you be sure that a plant has the best possibility of managing through disease and climatic variations? There can be great differences in the nutriment demands a plant places, all according to whether it is a cucumber, carrot or cabbage. Even the same plant naturally places different demands all according to its stage of development. A newly sprouted celery, for example, will die if it is exposed to the same nitrogen concentration as will make it grow optimally later in the season.

The ratio between the nutrients often plays just as great a role as the nutrients themselves. For example, a high content of iron and aluminum will prevent assimilation of phosphorus at low pH, and by adding lime phosphorus again becomes accessible.

A practical example familiar to most people is that a newly purchased flowering potted plant begins to "droop" even though it has plenty of water. The diagnosis is correct, however: the plant is dying of thirst. Because of lacking soil and the excessive addition of nutrients, the plant's roots are unable to absorb water. The plant dies from lack of water while simultaneously its "feet" are standing in water.

Symbiosis is a very important phenomenon in connection with plant nutrition, systems of cultivation and plant health. It is now known of many plant species that it is vitally necessary for them to live in a symbiosis, an intimate coexistence with one or several species of microorganisms.

Mycorrhiza are fungus hyphae which enter into a symbiosis with the plant's roots. The fungus obtains products from the plant's photosynthesis, and in return the plant receives, among other things, phosphorus, copper and zink, substances that all exist in combination with the soil and therefore are of difficult accessibility to the plant alone.

It has gradually become apparent that it is more the rule than the exception that plants live in symbiosis with these fungi. Many species, particularly trees, orchids and moorland plants, are completely dependent on the symbiosis, and if the fungus is not present in the soil the plants cannot grow. Plants having a coarse root system, for example onions, celery and leeks, grow very poorly without the symbiosis, while plants with a finer root system like grasses are much less dependent.

Many experiments show that plants manage better both under nutritive stress and attacks of disease when they live in symbiosis with mycorrhiza.

Leguminous plants' symbiosis with the nitrogen fixing rhizobium bacteria is one of the most well-known and important forms of symbiosis, from the viewpoint of an ecological system of cultivation. The bacteria form nodules on the roots of leguminous plants and fix atmospheric nitrogen. If the nitrogen level in the soil is high, the fixing of nitrogen from the air ceases. In terms of nitrogen pollution, nature thus has a built-in self-regulating safeguard.

This gives an idea of the many individual interactions that make it difficult, perhaps scientifically impossible, to determine a plant's optimum nutrient requirement at a given point in time.

Conditions of Cultivation

On the other hand, in Denmark, nearly all cucumbers and tomatoes are cultivated in soilless greenhouses in an inactive growth medium such as rock wool with the addition of 10-12 macro- and micronutrients. In Holland, around 40% of all vegetables are cultivated in this manner. When these substances are added the vegetables are supplied with all the substances that are necessary for the plant to grow as rapidly as possible. But what about all the other substances which plants have had access to from time immemorial, when they are cultivated the way plants, after all, always have been cultivated?

The industrial plants look like "healthy and robust" plants, but that is exclusively due to the fact that they are protected against attacks of disease. The plants' defense system is so miserable that here the term plant protection in connection with spray agents comes into its own. Preventive combat is necessary in order to avoid epidemics. The plants do not smell or taste like much, but the crops are hardly distinguishable from the vegetables humans have lived on for milleniums. So in a way there is no problem growing plants with few nutrients and apparently with tremendous results. On the other hand, the heads of lettuce, cucumbers and tomatoes we eat as the healthy daily supplement throughout the winter are an industrial product with a structure and a composition which are unknown to us. These crops never contain other substances than those added artificially. This means that the vegetable comes to lack many of the substances that are normally found in the soil and that for milleniums have been a natural part of the nutrients the plant absorbs. In all probability, it is only a small portion of these substances that we know the significance of today, which makes it even more alarming that we are changing the composition of especially that part of our diet that is supposed to constitute the healthy counterbalance to all of the foreign and, in part, toxic substances we ingest and surround ourselves with.

Parallel to the synthetically fed greenhouse crops, in the 1950s experiments were carried out on rats and mice, feeding experiments which at the time nobody assigned any special significance. The animals were fed a diet that contained all of the nutrients that were necessary, in synthetic form. And the animals thrived perfectly, just like the perfect head of lettuce. But if they were given carcinogenic substances, they developed many more tumors than the control animals which got normally cultivated feed.

From industrially produced greenhouse vegetables to the conventionally produced farm crops is not such a great qualitative leap as one might first believe.

The crops are grown in soil, to be sure, but with the addition of macro- and micronutrients in the form of fertilizers. In this way the plants receive all of the substances known that the crops in question must have, so as to be able to give as large a yield as possible.

The soil is used as a growth medium, and the suitability of the soil for retaining water and nutrients is essential. The fertility of the soil, however, is of minor significance as the plants are supplied with the nutrients that are necessary. The plants become large but weak and therefore, just as in the case of the greenhouse crops, have to be protected against weeds, insects and microorganisms with the aid of herbicides and pesticides.

In clear contrast to this is ecological and biodynamic farming, in which the basis for plant cultivation is the soil. The soil's fertility is the foundation and is all-decisive for the growth and health of the crops. The soil is manured as comprehensively as possible, and preferrably with composted biological material. From this great wealth and diversity of substances and potentials for entering into symbioses, the plants obtain the optimum conditions – not for maximum yield but for being able to hold their own as best possible under the varying environmental conditions, both with respect to climate, cultivation and disease.

There have been considerable comparative feeding experiments carried out on animals to see whether there were decisive differences in ecologically and conventionally grown feed. A number of experiments show that ecological feed has a greater biological value (Velimirov et al 1992), while others point to a connection between crops cultivated intensively using fertilizers and pesticides and reproductive disorders (Aehnelt & Hahn 1973, Plochberger 1989, Steiger 1986).

As early as around 1930 it was known that when animals are offered feed grown ecologically and with fertilizers, the animals, with great certainty, prefer the former. It would appear that the animals avoid as long as possible eating the feed cultivated with fertilizers. Ecological farmers can corroborate that if they have to feed with feeds that come from artificially fertilized fields, immediate problems arise in the form of refusal to eat and suddenly appearing sicknesses. Nobody disputes these observations' correctness, and a number of animal experiments likewise bear out the observations (Plochberger 1992). It seems that people have merely elected to disregard them.

That there can be decisive differences between two kinds of feed, which with respect to analysis contain the same nutrients in corresponding quantities, is very simply impossible to explain within present scientific reality. And it is no doubt mostly for that reason that people close their eyes to it (Levnedsmiddelstyrelsen 1990).

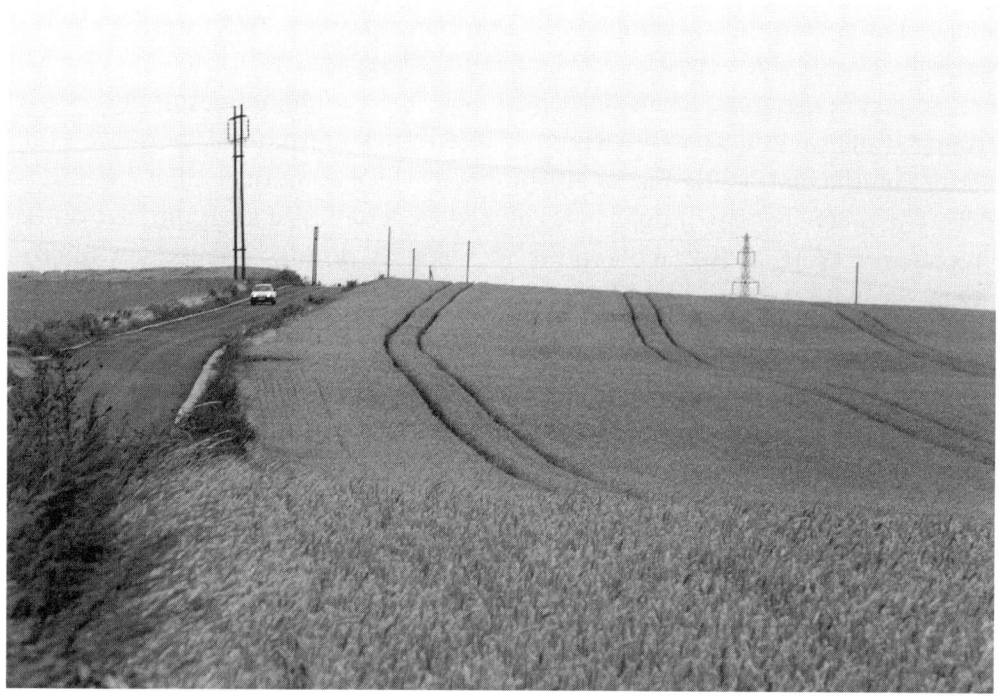

Weeds – Struggle or Dialogue

Within conventional farming weeds are viewed the way cancer is viewed within conventional medicine. Weeds are wild plants that grow in places we do not want them to be. They take light, water and nourishment from our crops, and they are unsightly – psychologically at any rate – in our ornamental beds. In our conventional way of thinking weeds are unwanted.

Conventionally, you spray weeds away with various agents, and if you are more ecologically minded you settle for burning, harrowing or chopping them. But they have got to go.

Instead of carrying on a struggle, a struggle we are doomed beforehand to lose, then opt for dialog. What is the story being told about the state and inner life of the soil when only some seeds sprout while others remain in a status of rest? Why do kinds of knotgrass grow in waterlogged soil, broom on lime-deficient land, stinging nettle in nutrient-rich soil and pansy in poor soil? Why do rhizobia bacteria cease fixing atmospheric nitrogen for the leguminous plant when the nitrogen level in the soil exceeds a certain level? And why do fungi only form sclerotia – stores of nourishment in the mycellia – when the soil is poor?

Up until now we have chosen the struggle as the explicatory model. The Darwinistic model in which the strong survives. The best adapted outcompetes the others.

You could chose another model. You could understand the calcium aggregates on the broom's roots as a way the broom compensates for the soil's lacking lime content. And you could view in the same manner the ability of the knotgrass in waterlogged soil to absorb water and let it evaporate, and the ability of fungi in poor soils to form sclerotia. This means that specific species contribute to balancing the soil, and by removing weeds we are contributing to making the imbalance even greater. On that background it is possible to understand the different species' presence as a language, the soil's language. A language whereby the soil can signal what state it is in, what it lacks and what there is too much of. A rich and varied language will in that connection be an expression of a healthier and more living soil than a soil which only has few species – an impoverished and less varied language.

Against that background, a great diversity will not only signal the possibility of a more living soil. An investigation done by Hald and Reddersen in 1990 (Miljøministeriet 1990) also reveals that there are many more species of plants in ecologically cultivated fields than in those cultivated conventionally, and which, it should be noted parenthetically, were for experimental reasons not sprayed with pesticides while the investigations were going on. A monoculture field sprayed for weeds will therefore have a tendency to create greater imbalances than an ecologically cultivated field.

On account of their deeper roots, trees can signal a more deep-seated language than the herbaceous plants can. Along an avenue it is very often seen that the treetops vary in height in a systematic way. The trees standing across from each other are very alike, and an undulating line is formed when the treetops down along the avenue are connected. The state of the soil at that level corresponds rather to the person's innate qualities or handicaps, all according to who the observer is. It means that it is much more difficult to do anything about this imbalance, in most cases very likely impossible.

Health, Quality and Language

Within conventional farming and market gardening, plant and animal health is experienced as the absence of diseases, or simply diseases that cannot be known. By way of example, the difference between the dark and dry pork and normal pork is naturally not so simple that it is a mere question of more or less lactic acid. The living organism does not function as simply as a machine. If displacements occur in one area of the living organism, there will also occur displacements in the chemical conditions in a series of other areas. If the chemical and biological displacements are serious, there is thus also reason to ask whether the meat is fit for human consumption.

A greenhouse cucumber is experienced as healthy and sound because it has been prophylactically sprayed and therefore has not gotten sick from a pathogenic fungus attack. But is it? What does this sickness/health concept mean for the quality of our foodstuffs?

In the conventional way of thinking, high foodstuff quality has to fulfill basically two requirements: the foodstuffs must contain adequate amounts of nutritious matter – theoretically we could ingest our food synthetically in pill form – and the foodstuffs must not contain toxic substances in such large quantities that it is possible in the short term to find linkages between the substance in question and sicknesses. We are speaking primarily of substances like heavy metals, pesticides, mycotoxins, nitrate and antibiotics. In this line of reasoning sprayed crops and antibiotics-fed livestock can therefore be healthy. In the present health model, foodstuffs which have either been irradiated or microwave treated will therefore often be of a better quality than foodstuffs without these treatments. Irradiated foodstuffs probably contain fewer pathogenic fungus spores, and microwave treatment preserves a higher content of certain vitamins. For the many sciences which do not reckon with other than purely material physical and chemical factors, such a concept of quality is self-evident, indeed so self-evident that it is perceived, not as philosophical theory, but as fact.

Ethics and the Scientific Paradigm

Surprisingly many parallels can be drawn between states in human beings, animals, plants and the soil. In the following I will illustrate this.

If living organisms are subjected to stress, having to yield, produce, work too much over an extended period, the organism responds by going into a state of stress and lack of well-being. If the state persists, sicknesses arise.

Within the past few years, when we in Denmark have had several mild winters in a row, it has been possible to observe evergreen trees and shrubs that have died after having over a series of years shown an increasing number of brown leaves and needles. They are suffering from stress – overexertion from not having obtained the needed rest during the winter months that is normal for them. The absence of low winter temperatures has meant that photosynthesis, and with it the other life processes, have not been reduced to the same extent as is normal for Danish acclimatized plants. Even plants need to rest.

We do not have a language to describe the state we are in when we seek out the doctor on account of lack of well-being, and neither the doctor nor the health system at large is able to register anything abnormal. This is the state by far the predominant part of our foodstuffs are and have been in for the past forty to fifty years. One wonders what impact it has had on the state of human health that we have been living on food which can be apprehended as being healthy only for want of concepts.

We are many scientific investigators who, in spite of intellectually knowing very well that everything in the world cannot be reduced to analysable inert things, must nevertheless, by virtue of our methods, reduce everything to manipulable physical and chemical quantities. Modern man is split in two. In our jobs we observe rules and not our hearts, and the dilemma arises: the ethical aspect is excluded. Even if this appears to be a fact, it is certainly not a Law of Nature. The great ethical and, up through the eighties and nineties, political questions, like euthanasia, test-tube babies, genetic manipulation, organ transplantation and the nonviable premature infant, we are unable to deal with ethically, as long as we think and act quantitatively and reducibly.

If the sciences are to seriously have any meaning they must throw light on our lives and relations. Scientific insight must not be reduced to only dealing with inert things, and a scientist must not be reduced to being an objective and anonymous spectator. Gradually, it is dawning on us that the scientific results, which through hundreds of years we have produced on the notion that science is a storyless, objective, anonymous observation of and manipulation of chemical and physical facts, are an illusion. For many scientists this view still appears so self-evident that they cannot even catch sight of the fact that their way of dealing with science is theoretical and nothing else. Naturally, this is because the sciences have had the dominant role in the creation of our material welfare.

Conclusion

Are the increasing patronage of the alternative medicine network and augmented demand for ecologically produced foodstuffs mere fads and entirely fortuitous?

There are many signs that a development is underway, a development which has its roots in a stronger development of the individual, and in a greater awareness of widespread social and global problems.

Increased social welfare and security have contributed to making us blind to the undesirable aspects of the growth society. But as the drawbacks have come into view, awareness has increased and our identity has become sharper.

The failure of the established health services in the face of a growing number of illnesses, and a medical treatment that is mechanical and devoid of subject, has no doubt been essential for making visible the lopsidedness of conventional agriculture, and for the evolvement of ecological farming. There are many similarities between the alternative health services and ecological farming's conception and view of health, the treatment of illness and the whole concept of the individual. The same concord can manifest itself even across professional boundaries when it is a question of moral and ethical norms, attitudes towards nature and the entire world view (Kaltoft 1996). Attitudes are associated with an awareness of the fact that problems with respect to environment and disease are intimately connected with the reductionistic outlook of established society, and cannot be solved through continued growth. Even within the same discipline this understanding can, for reasons of attitude and awareness, be so great that a dialogue is impossible.

References

Aehnelt, E. & Hahn, J.
1973   "Fruchtbarkeit der Tiere – eine Möglichkeit zur biologischen Qualitätsprüfung von Futter und Nahrungsmitteln?", in: *Tierärztliche Umschau*, 28: 155-160.

Andreasen, Chr. & Jensen, J. E.
1994   "11. Danske Planteværnskonference i Ukrudt: Herbicidresistens i Danmark", in: *SP rapport*, 6: 261-270.

Bertrand, G.
1905   "Sur l'emplai favorable du manganèse comme engrais", in: *C. R. Acad. Sci. Paris*, 141: 1255.

Braun, U., et al.
1983   "Beziehungen zwischen Milchleistung, Milchzusammensetzung und Fruchtbarkeit bei Schweizer Braunviehkühen sowie Einfluß der Rastzeit auf das Erstbesamungsergebnis", in: *Schweizer Archiv für Tierheilkunde*, 125: 477-490.

de Cock, J., Westveer, K., Heederik, D., te Velde, E. & van Kooij, R.
1994   "Time to pregnancy and occupational exposure to pesticides in fruit growers in The Netherlands", in: *Occup. Environ. Med.*, 51: 693-699.

Hansen, N. & Hansen, D.
1978   "Degeneration og mangelsygdomme" in*: Mad – er ikke bare mad*, Forlag Borgen: Copenhagen.

Holt, J. S., Powles, S. B. and Holtum, J. A. M.
1993   "Mechanisms and agronomic aspects of herbicide resistance", in: *Annual Review of Plant Physiology and Plant Molecular Biology*, 44: 203-229.

Kaltoft, P.
1996   "Ingeniører og naturetik", in: *Miljøetik*, NSU series.

Landbrugs- og fiskeriministeriet
1995   *Aktionsplan for fremme af den økologiske fødevareproduktion i Danmark*, Landbrugs- og fiskeriministeriet.

Landbrugsrådet
1995   *Danske fødevarer frem mod år 2000*, Landbrugsrådet, sept. 1995.

Levnedsmiddelstyrelsen
1990   *Frugt og grøntsager vurderet udfra et helhedssyn.*

Margna, U., Margna, E. & Vainjärv, T.
1989   "Influence of nitrogen nutrition on the utilization of L-phenylalanine for building flavonoids in buckwheat seedling tissues", in: *J. Plant Physiol.*, 134: 697-702.

Miljø- og Energiministeriet
1995   *Natur- og Miljøpolitisk redegørelse 1995*, Miljø og Energiministeriet: Copenhagen.

Miljøministeriet
1990   *Fugleføde i kornmarker – insekter og vilde planter*, Miljøprojekt nr. 125, Miljøministeriet, Miljøstyrelsen.

Plochberger, K.
1989   "Feeding Experiments. A criterion for quality estimation of biologically and conventionally produced foods", in: *Agriculture, Ecosystems and Environment*, 27: 419-428.

Plochberger, K. & Velimirov, A.
1992   "Are food preference tests with laboratory rats proper method for evaluating nutritional quality?", in: *Biological Agriculture and Horticulture*, 8: 221-233.

Pounden, W. D. & Frank, N. A.
1961   "Influence of forages on mastitis", in: *J. Amer. Vet. Med. Ass.*, 138: 146-150.

Silverstone, H., Solomon, R. D., Tannenbaum, A.
1952   "Relative influences of natural and semipurified diets on tumor formation in mice", in: *Cancer Res.*, 12: 750-756.

Specialarbejderforbundet i Danmark
1995   *Rapport om økologisk jordbrugsreform*, Specialarbejderforbundet i Danmark, sept. 1995.

Steiger, D.
1986   *Einfluss konventionell und biologisch-dynamisch angebauten Futters auf Fruchtbarkeit, allgemeinen Gesundheitszustand und Fleischqualität beim Hauskaninchen*, Dissertation, Univ. Bonn.

Toldam-Andersen, T. & Hansen, P.
1995   "Source-sink relations in fruits. VIII. The effect of nitrogen on fruit/leaf-ratios and fruit development in apple", in: *Acta Horticulturae*, 383: 25-33.

Velimirov, A., Plochberger, K., Huspeka, U. & Schott, W.
1992   "The influence of biologically and conventionally cultivated food on the fertility of rats", in: *Biol. Agriculture and Horticulture*, 8: 325-337.

Woodward, J.
1699   "Some thoughts and experiments on vegetation", in: *Phil. Trans. Roy. Soc. London*, 21: 382.

Methodology, Methodology Abstracts, INRAT Evaluation

Methodologies along a Spectrum:

From the Randomized Controlled Trial to Post-Modern Queries

by Mary Ryan-Thorup

Methodologies and their value in designing projects for determining the benefits of alternative medicine have been a heated topic at every INRAT seminar. The last one was no exception. This paper presents the results of seminar discussions about what methodologies are relevant for alternative medical research. Different methodologies answer different questions, from the randomized controlled trial to more socio-cultural questions, such as who uses alternative medicine and why. Over the past four years, there has been a polarization of discussion between the biomedical methodology camp and the social. This is reflected in the abstracts that participants were invited to submit about methodological considerations in alternative medical research at the last INRAT seminar (see pages 181-204). To contextualise this discussion of methodologies, the motivation for undertaking research on alternative medicine is briefly mentioned first. The general aims of alternative medical research are also delineated to clarify the range of research questions being considered. Nine categories of methodologies are then presented. These categories represent the predominant themes in the abstracts written by participants, and also articles by contributors to the INRAT volumes I-III. By categorizing the different methodologies, discussions are clarified about who is researching what in relation to determining the benefits of a given alternative medical treatment.

Motivation

For the sake of clarity, it is important to delineate the various motivations for researching therapies and their use in Europe and abroad. The increased use of alternative medicine in Europe is well documented, as in Helle Johannessen's article (Johannessen 1994) and Hofmeister and colleagues' article (Hofmeister et al. 1994). The popular demand has reached such a high level that the dominant medical systems in Europe are required to look at what alternative therapy has to offer the general population in terms of efficacy. For alternative practitioners, there is the issue of gaining legitimacy in the eyes of the dominant political-economic medical establishment so that resources may be shared, thus supporting their ability to treat patients and conduct their own research. Thus, a dialogue is being forged between the biomedical establishment and the alternative therapy sector.

The general research aims with respect to alternative medical research are:

1) to measure the efficacy of alternative therapies from the scientific viewpoint, yet with respect for the alternative therapeutic criteria, i.e., compromising the double-blind, randomized, controlled trial.
2) to investigate principles of curing and healing purportedly used in alternative therapies.
3) to bring alternative therapies into the established healthcare system, thus gaining financial support, legitimation, standardisation and quality control for the benefit of users safety. (However, this is a controversial aim that not all researchers of alternative medical policy agree with).
4) to close the "credibility gap" between advocates of biomedicine and advocates of alternative medicine, and respective patients and users.

Methodology Categories

Abstracts were presented at the last INRAT seminar on the development of methodologies that clarify these different aims in alternative medical research. Nine different categories of methodologies were considered, inspired by these abstracts and previous articles written by participants in the INRAT Volumes 1-3, and other publications by the same authors. The nine methodology categories are concerned with determining the benefits of alternative therapies along a spectrum from the narrow, biomedical definition of efficacy, to broader forms of life quality, effectiveness and intrinsic value. The categories are:

1) measuring efficacy of an alternative treatment on the basis of a purely physiological definition;
2) measuring efficacy with quality of life methodologies;
3) physiotherapy measures, dealing with physical movement and its relation to task ability in the home;
4) intersubjective measures: experience related to everyday life from the perspectives of: patient satisfaction, family satisfaction, practitioner satisfaction.

5) financial: cost effectiveness;
6) political-economic concerns, such as place of alternative medicine within society;
7) cultural analysis, such as in the case of transplanting medical systems from other cultures, and the implication and also understanding principles of health and treatment outcome from the perspective of another culture's medical system;
8) ecological analysis, such as the environmental effects of both biomedical and alternative medical research, and the effects of pesticides on general health;
9) aesthetic evaluation of alternative therapies, such as their intrinsic, felt value that goes beyond measurement.

These categories represent a summary of research methodology interests written by authors that contributed to the INRAT volumes 1-3, *Studies in Alternative Therapy*. While it would be exhaustive to report on every aspect of the topic of methodologies and alternative therapies, each author that writes about methodology is listed below for further reference.

In category one, various authors wrote about the methodology of measuring the efficacy of an alternative therapy from a purely physiological definition, including the randomized controlled trial. The authors are: Robert Anderson (see this volume) Toke Barfod (This volume and Book Three), Christian Borchgrevink (This volume and Book One), Stig Bruset (Book One), Leila Eriksen (Book One), Renate Hoffmann-Dorninger (Book Two), Laila Launsø (see this volume), Dieter Melchart (Book One), Phillip Nicholls (This volume and Book Two), Rebecca Rees (Book Three), Bruno Riek (see this volume) and Wolfgang Weidenhammer (see this volume).

In category two, 8 authors mentioned measuring the efficacy of alternative therapies using quality of life measures. The authors are: Robert Anderson (see this volume), Toke Barfod (see this volume), Stig Bruset (Book One), Leila Eriksen (Book One), Renate Hoffmann-Dorninger (book Two), Gunnar Johansson (Book One), Laila Launsø (see this volume) and Phillip Nicholls (Book Two).

In category three, physiotherapy measures, three authors mentioned the use of this methodology. The authors are: Stig Bruset (Book One), Leila Eriksen (Book One) and Mary Ryan-Thorup (Book Three).

In category four, intersubjective measures, such as patient and practitioner satisfaction, 14 authors discussed this methodology. The authors are: David Aldridge (Book Two), Robert Anderson (see this volume), Christian Borchgrevink (Book One), Eva Brendstrup (Book One), Leila Eriksen (Book One), Erlendur Haraldsson (Book One), Renate Hoffmann-Dorninger (Book Two),

Elsebeth Hofmeister, et al. (Book One), Elisabeth Hsu (Book Three), Dieter Melchart (Book Three), Phillip Nicholls (Book Two), Rebecca Rees (Book Three), Bruno Riek (see this volume) and Ursula Sharma (Book Two).

In category five, cost effectiveness, authors have discussed the importance of determining cost effectiveness of alternative treatments. The authors are Robert Anderson (see this volume), Phillip Nicholls (see this volume and Book Two) and Stig Bruset (Book One).

In category six, political-economic concerns, the following authors have addressed this issue: Robert Anderson (see this volume), Phillip Nicholls (see this volume and Book Two) and Espen Braathen (Book Three).

In category seven, cultural analysis, many authors have written about cultural implications of the development and spread of various alternative medical systems. The authors are: Motzi Eklöf (Book Three), Stephen Fulder (Book Two), Helle Johannessen (Book Three), Phillip Nicholls (Book Two), Ib Lundgaard Rasmussen (Book Two), Ursula Sharma (Books Two and Three), and James Spickard (Book Two).

In category eight, ecological analysis, while many participants at the seminars brought up the importance of this category, very little has been written about it. However, Laila Launsø (see this volume) and Kirsten Skjerbæk (see this volume) have begun to address this concern.

In category nine, aesthetic evaluation of alternative therapies, the following authors have written: Jørgen Østergård Andersen (see this volume), Renate Hoffmann-Dorninger (Book Two), Laila Launsø (see this volume), Meredith McGuire (Book Two), Hjördis Nerheim (see this volume), Søren Gosvig Olesen (Book Two), and Kirsten Skjerbæk (see this volume).

Abstract Session

The abstract session at the last seminar that discussed these methodology categories was inspiring: it was agreed that no one methodology had all the answers. The only way forward is through mutual recognition of the knowledge gained from each methodology. It was agreed that through the integration of different methodologies a more subtle understanding could be obtained of the benefits of given alternative treatments. As stated by Helle Johannessen in her abstract:

> "It should be obvious that different conceptual constructions of disease and healing call for different kinds of evaluation, and that several methods can supplement each other in a methodology including one and the other research method...Much would be gained, if we stopped

arguing what method is the Right One. The simple answer is: None of them alone – but all of them together. Supplementing each other's qualitative and quantitative research may provide an estimation of a variety of 'values' and 'qualities' of a given form of treatment. A complex [of methodologies] may reveal 'significance' of this treatment in several aspects: for the patient (physically, socially, emotionally and culturally), for the practitioner, for society, and for nature...." (Johannessen, this volume: 191).

Phillip Nicholls in his abstract and discussion group echoed this idea, and qualified the categorisation of the different methodologies. These methodologies differ from one another in outcome. The challenge in alternative medical research is not to decide on one unified methodology, but to preserve the diversity of approaches. The importance of dialogue and openness between medical and social research groups should be stressed. This discussion also centred around the distinction between efficacy and effectiveness. Efficacy in the biomedical realm is concerned with physiological and biochemical test outcome in controlled trials. Effectiveness is also concerned with outcome but is described instead in terms of the patient-practitioner interaction, and qualitative effectiveness from the patient's personal viewpoint. The difference between efficacy and effectiveness is that outcome is measured in different *settings* and with different *parameters*. Laila Launsø in her abstract also made this point:

"We are researching a field where treatments cannot be standardised but must be adapted to the individual. The situation calls for the development of a 'science of the unique or the concrete', that is 'context dependent science' including the treatment model, the concrete treatment approach and effects defined in a very broad way...." (Launsø, this volume: 193).

This discussion group also focused on the resulting importance of the social science researcher who is able to distinguish between different methodologies and their underlying assumptions, and can act as a communication link between the different groups.

The Intersection of Biomedicine and the Social Sciences

In the past, the health sciences have been divided into two branches, the biological and the behavioral or social. It became obvious from reading the contributions to the INRAT books, Volumes One, Two and Three, that researchers either took a biological or a behavioral social stance when discussing alternative medicine and how to apply methodologies to determine their benefits. The purpose of this section is to orient this discussion about methodologies and alternative medicine within the larger debate of the intersection of the biological and social sciences. We are now moving into a new era of research, where these domains are no longer so divided. By seeing where, methodologically, the intersection takes place between biomedicine and the social sciences, we can better understand the place of our research on determining the effectiveness of alternative medicine from various perspectives.

Lola Romanucci-Ross, et al. give an instructive example of the paradigmatic extremes of biological and social thought and how they can view the same situation quite differently. The biomedical paradigm tells us that tuberculosis is caused by *Myobacterium tuberculosis*, whereas the behavioral science paradigm tells us that tuberculosis is "caused" by poverty and malnutrition. The attitude that people take toward a condition such as tuberculosis, and its physically observable symptoms (such as loss of breath, rattling sound in the throat when breathing, coughing, and lethargy) is shaped by culture. Culture can be broadly defined as "the system of meaning – belief knowledge and action – by which people organize their lives" (Romanucci-Ross 1991). This behavioral organization also determines the diseases to which people are subject, and which medical system they choose to alleviate their condition. To understand different sicknesses people have, the choices in health care they are making, and the benefits of possible treatments available, we must begin with the underlying cosmologies and principles of healing of the various medical systems, and also the underlying cosmologies of the patients choosing them. Elisabeth Hsu in her abstract raised this point:

> "What do people [practitioners and patients] talk about who speak of auras, prana, qi, etc.? Does treatment evaluation of alternative therapies have to take account of their conceptualisation of man and the universe and the language they use to speak about it? Why bother to understand these languages for treatment evaluation?" (Hsu, this volume: 190).

This adds an important dimension to research on alternative medical treatments. Each study undertaken to discover the efficacy, effectiveness and general benefits of a given alternative treatment will contain greater or lesser components of the biological and socio-cultural paradigms. The importance of both perspectives is becoming more recognised now in both biomedical and social circles. Each is useful in varying degrees, depending upon the therapy under investigation.

Critique of Biomedicine

The past two decades have witnessed a growing critique of biomedicine within the social sciences, and even in biomedical circles as well. Since this criticism is inherent in many of the abstracts, it is important to clarify what it is about biomedicine that social researchers criticize. Foucault is well known for his critique of biomedicine in *The Birth of a Clinic* (1975), where he states that the body became an object of social control with the spread of the industrial revolution and capitalism. Bodies, individuals, were minutely observed in factories, classrooms, clinics, prisons, and hospitals. Bodies were made into docile instruments for use in the exercise of economic and political power. Along with this increase in power over individuals came the birth of the dossier, of collections of documents about populations on a large scale, in terms of health, economic welfare, education, etc. This type of documentation led to the "case study," to the creation of "subjects" and "numbers" isolated from their social background and personal lives.

Similarly, in the work of Michael Taussig, (1980), a hospitalized patient is described who is convinced of her own helplessness in the face of disease. She minimises her own strength because she has been taught to rely on experts who function to invalidate her intuitive understanding of the social origin of her problem. Her disease is treated as a thing, part of a natural world separate from the social world that oppresses her. Taussig considers biomedicine to express a hidden ideology that reifies the social and separates it into a natural domain where it cannot be understood for what it is. By placing the body and the bodily experience in the realm of nature, biomedicine can conceal the social causes of sickness, and the social embeddedness of the experience of being sick (Rhodes 1990). The danger in biomedicine is that its posture of factuality is precisely its power: value-neutral language can neutralize who we are when we are sick, and neutralize the greater social event of sickness. Here it is important to acknowledge the work of Laila Launsø, in which she has defined this problem as the scope of diagnosis and the user's scope of action: the narrower the scope of diagnosis, the smaller the scope of action available to the patient (Launsø, this volume: 136).

Researchers in biomedical fields are themselves facing this dilemma. Biomedicine is expanding its definitions of physical disorder, incorporating problems with recognizably larger social components (for example, alcoholism, posttraumatic stress disorder), and recognizing the way that psychological stress can lead to physical imbalances.

As the dominant political and economic medical power, biomedical institutions also control the use of and research into alternative medicine. Yet biomedicine fails to provide means for alternative types of treatments to "prove" themselves. It should be noted that this is not a failure of science, but a failure of the medical establishment's methodological tools. The goal of the scientific method is to be non-authoritative: to provide methods which give everyone a chance to prove themselves. Alternative medicine thus poses a great methodological challenge.

Critique of Social Science

Social science researchers are not without their own Cartesian dualism and reductionist tendencies. Social scientists need to look at the limitations of their own discipline also. Disease and illness, for example, present a well known distinction that has been useful in the delineation of biological versus social issues in efficacy research. This distinction is based upon dividing up the field of "sickness" into a domain of disease, considered to be pathology as medically defined, and illness, which encompasses all the cultural, social implications of sickness experienced by the patient.

What has happened in many efficacy studies undertaken by sociologists and anthropologists is that the disease part of the sickness picture has been left out, and the focus turned to understanding illness. This also can delegitimize the experience of patients, by seeing all their problems as due to social events and larger macrosocial and spiritual struggles that are removed from the reality of having, say, cancer. This has also meant that many social scientists have studied the social implications of sickness in medical settings, often ignoring the fact that the disease half of the picture is itself a cultural construction that deserves explanation. As pointed out by Lorna Rhodes, it is important to study groups of patients suffering from a particular disease and the relationship between cultural and physical aspects of causation in a particular disorder, in ways that are relevant to the social context supporting the research (Rhodes 1990). This has further been indicated by Noel Chrisman and Thomas Maretzki, where they state: *"In our research, anthropologists have explicitly or implicitly drawn on clinical medicine as the standard for judging the 'real' world of sickness"* (Chrisman and Maretzki 1982: 22).

Being accessories in this work in medical settings, and in the disease/illness dichotomy, anthropologists might fall into the same Cartesian trap of the mind-body dualism, for which biomedicine is being criticized (Hahn 1984). By using the disease/illness distinction, by separating nature from culture, social scientists run the same risks of taking on the same characteristics of the biomedical advocates they are fond of criticizing (Rhodes 1990).

The Role of the Observer

Social science is also facing the breaking of its foundations: there is an emergence now of new paradigms that are attempting to move away from the bounded subject and object of ethnographic research. The attempt is to think interactively, in dialogues. This shift brings great hope for methodological issues in efficacy research. This move is toward what Michael Jackson has called "lived experience" (1989). Lived experience, in his view, has more to do with the flow between subject and object, the interplay and dialectical relationship between ethnographer and informants. It stresses the "participation" in participant observation methodologies in social science, and involves acknowledging more clearly the positionality of knowledge that is expressed in fieldwork. Through admitting our "bias," and the perspective of the observer/researcher, a new domain of knowledge is apprehended, creating dialogues between observer, practitioner, patient, with clear communication between the different worlds, giving to social research a living, dynamic quality.

Michael Jackson claims we can ground our personal experiences in fieldwork with the Other as a reflection and part of ourselves (rather than an isolated, different Other). The method of doing this kind of fieldwork is termed "radical empiricism," and is a way of grounding interpersonal experience in social research based upon the early 20th century writing of William James (1912). Radical empiricism can be applied in social science as an experience of objects and action in which the subject itself is a participant (Jackson citing Edie 1989: 12), admitting the personal subjective experience as part of the many perspectives drawn on in social research. This gives more movement and *opportunities for exchange through time* during research. This new movement in social research was reflected also in Laila Launsø's abstract where she stated:

> "...different modes of research produce different types of knowledge and represent different knowledge systems. The descriptive and explanatory modes of research produce objectivistic knowledge; the understanding mode of research produces hermeneutic knowledge and the action-oriented mode of research produces praxeological knowledge. In order to understand healing processes, we need to give priority to produce knowledge related to understanding and action-oriented research" (Launsø, this volume: 193).

It also means the researcher is no longer a static, objective observer, but is both observer and participator. William James writes: *"Our fields of experience have no more definite boundaries than our fields of view. Both are fringed for-*

ever by a more *that continuously develops, and that continuously supersedes them as life proceeds"* (James 1976: 35). The "self" then – of the researcher or the patient or the clinician – is not seen as a *"thing among things; it is a function of our involvement with others in a world of diverse and ever-altering interests and situations"* (Jackson 1989). Jørgen Østergård Andersen touched on exactly this point in his abstract, Aesthetic Evaluation of Alternative Therapies:

> "The patient, who is disturbed and uncomfortable, and when he or she is confronted with a painful experience or memory...is not in a position to evaluate the intervention of the therapist, who is not in a position to evaluate his own intervention. The therapist can only legitimise his own practise, and by reference to a theoretical system the therapist may want to share the responsibility of his or her intervention with a collectivity; but only a third part (to the relationship between the therapist and the patient) can evaluate the outcome of a treatment – and only by a criterion which is aesthetic...Only a third part is in a position to see, to judge and to appreciate whether an intervention is necessary or not, whether the style of the therapist is beautiful or ugly...Such an evaluation is a matter of taste of the observer of course, but it is wrong to think that a taste is something personal. We share a taste with others, and therefore it is not impossible to evaluate the outcome of a therapy [aesthetically], but an evaluation and a judgement must be negotiated by the collective which shares the taste" (Andersen, this volume: 181).

The importance of this approach is that the focus in social research is changed from the observer and the observed to the *interplay* between the observer and the observed. The focus is on processual knowledge. Boundaries are dropped between individuals, and yet retained with flexibility through direct communication across fields of knowing. This approach is useful also in the broader field of methodological research because determining the benefits of alternative medicine requires that we talk across subdisciplines. It sees everyone as an accessary and involved in the evolution of health research strategies. It admits to the connectedness of the different disciplines involved in health research, and helps us to admit that we are all involved along a continuum of time filled with both revelations and unanswered questions.

Building Bridges of Mutual Recognition

Being sick entails an intensity, vulnerability and suffering that reveals attitudes and reactions in the society in which it occurs. Sickness throws into relief issues and contradictions that are not so evident when there is less at stake (Kleinman 1988). When sick people are faced with the fact that biomedicine is not working for them, the foundations of knowledge and security begin to crumble under them, and they are faced with creating a new foundation by seeking healing from other medical systems and their practitioners.

Our society is also sick: the ecological destruction of the planet, pollution, widespread poverty and malnutrition contrasted to the incredible wealth of a few individuals does not represent a highly evolved species. In the established medical systems of Europe and even in the developing nations, there are symptoms of the crumbling foundations of present economic, social and scientific systems of thought. Within biomedicine, its practitioners are acutely aware that reductionism is not working: the importance of a larger framework is becoming increasingly, painfully evident. This pain and vulnerability of our selves, of the body, of our societies, even of the alternative and biomedical establishments that recognize that they do not have all the answers: this pain is evident and is what makes debates about biomedicine versus alternative medicine so heated.

How one thinks about biomedicine makes a difference in how one approaches efficacy and creating methodologies to determine the benefits (and adverse effects) of alternative treatments. As biomedical doctors, researchers, as practitioners and as social scientists all involved in alternative medical research, we must face the fact that the dominant medical-political power in the West is biomedicine. Indeed, its principles of practise are breaking apart and in need of restructuring. But still, there are no alternative medical practitioners on medical research funding boards in Europe. It is important to orient research aims toward interdisciplinary research that includes even the biomedical establishment. By clearly defining one's role and relationship to biomedicine – the dominant medical political establishment in the West – understanding about different methodologies and how they are to be applied in alternative medical research is easier. Ultimately, researchers of alternative medicine are in the same position as clinicians: to be of service and to contribute to the alleviation of suffering.

It is also necessary to appreciate the strength of biomedicine, despite its many limitations. Researchers in biomedicine are faced with the difficult task of determining what treatments are to be made available to the public. If these researchers make a mistake, discarding a treatment that should not have been discarded, or accepting a treatment that should not have been accepted, it may be a matter of life and death for many people. The responsibility is tremendous, and is also another reason for the intensity of the struggle between biomedical researchers and social scientists to find suitable criteria for determining whether or not a treatment "works."

The researchers that have networked through INRAT these past four years have been communicating across methodological paradigms. In concluding this time of dialogue, the "objectivist" position still dominates efficacy and health status research. However, various research (cf. Anderson this volume; Melchart 1996; Ryan 1996) has shown the benefits of complementing objective, biomedical research with intersubjective viewpoints.

References

Chrisman, Noel and Thomas J. Maretzki
1982   *Clinically Applied Anthropology: Anthropologists in Health Science Settings*, D. Reidel: Dordrecht.

Foucault, Michel
1975   *The Birth of a Clinic: An Archaeology of Medical Perception*, Vintage: New York.

Hahn, Robert A.
1984   "Rethinking illness and disease", in: *Contributions to Asian Studies*, 18(1): 23.

Hofmeister, Elsebeth et al.
1994   "Centers for integrated medicine in Denmark: Explanatory models for disease, treatment methods, modes of practise and users", in: Johannessen, Helle, Laila Launsø, Søren Gosvig Olesen and Frants Staugård (eds.): *Studies in Alternative Therapy 1 – Contributions from the Nordic Countries*, Odense University Press: Odense.

Jackson, Michael
1988   *Paths Toward a Clearing: Radical Empiricism and Ethnographic Enquiry*, pp. 1-18, Indiana University Press: Bloomington and Indianapolis.

Johannessen, Helle, Launsø, Laila, Olesen, Søren Gosvig & Staugård Frants (eds.)
1994   *Studies in Alternative Therapy 1. Contributions from the Nordic Countries*, Odense University Press: Odense.

Johannessen, Helle, Olesen, Søren Gosvig & Andersen, Jørgen Østergård (eds.)
1995   *Studies in Alternative Therapy 2. Body and Nature*, Odense University Press: Odense.

Kleinman, Arthur M.
1988   *The Illness Narratives*, Basic Books: New York.

Melchart, Dieter
1996   "Integration of Complementary Medicine in Research at the University of Munich", in: Søren Gosvig Olesen and Erling Høg (eds.): *Studies in Alternative Therapy 3. Communication in and about Alternative Therapies*, pp. 159-170, Odense University Press: Odense.

Olesen, Søren Gosvig & Høg, Erling (eds.)
1996   *Studies in Alternative Therapy 3. Communication in and about Alternative Therapies*, Odense University Press: Odense.

Rhodes, Lorna Amarasingham
1990   "Studying biomedicine as a cultural system", in: Thomas M. Johnson and Carolyn F. Sargent (eds.): *Medical Anthropology: Contemporary Theory and Method*, Praeger: New York.

Romanucci-Ross, Lola, Daniel Moerman, and Laurence Tancredi
1994   *The Anthropology of Medicine: From Culture to Method*, Bergin and Garvey: New York.

Ryan, Mary
1996   *Using Multiple Methodologies to Measure Cross-Cultural Efficacy: The Tibetan Medical Treatment for Arthritis*, PhD Dissertation, Bodleian Library, Oxford University.

Taussig, Michael
1980   "Reification and the consciousness of the patient", in: *Social Science and Medicine*, 14 B: 3-13.

Aesthetic Evaluation of Alternative Therapies

by Jørgen Østergård Andersen

How do we define or measure the efficacy of alternative therapies like psychotherapy (for instance psychoanalysis, group therapy, family therapy and gestalt therapy) and spiritual healing (for instance meditation and prayers), and how do we measure the therapeutic outcome of human potential groups, energy exercises etc.?

An easy answer to the question – and a correct one – is that we cannot measure the efficacy of such kinds of treatments, since the therapeutic outcome is not comparable to the outcome of an allopathic treatment. We have only a very limited perspective on alternative therapies, if they are merely perceived as a duplication of conventional medicine. The outcome of such therapies is not an efficacy, which is measurable.

This does not imply, however, that such therapies cannot be evaluated and that a therapeutic treatment – like a therapeutic session – cannot be evaluated. It is obvious that some sessions are better – or more "effective" than other sessions. The quality of two therapists and of two different therapeutic sessions are never the same. How can we expose this difference, and how can we appreciate a treatment which is helpful to a patient, and criticize another treatment which may be harmful to a patient, when the criterion for such an evaluation is difficult – or impossible – to establish?

The patient who is disturbed and uncomfortable when he or she is confronted with a painful experience or memory (from childhood for instance), is not in a position to evaluate the intervention of the therapist, who is not in a position to evaluate his own intervention. The therapist can only legitimize his own practice, and by reference to a theoretical system the therapist may want to share the responsibility of his or her intervention with a collectivity; but only a third part (to the relationship between the therapist and the patient) can evaluate the outcome of a treatment – and only by a criterion which is aesthetic.

Only a third part is in an position to see, judge and appreciate whether an intervention is necessary or not, whether the style of performance of the therapist is beautiful or ugly or whether the outcome of the session is good or bad. Such an evaluation is a matter of the taste of the observer, of course, but it is wrong to think that taste is something personal. We share taste with others, and therefore it is not impossible to evaluate the outcome of a therapy, but an evaluation and a judgement must be negotiated by the collectivity which shares the taste.

It is an illusion that the efficacy of a therapeutic intervention can be measured, and it is wrong to believe that the result of measurements say anything meaningful about the therapeutic outcome of alternative therapies like psychotherapy, meditation, spiritual healing, body therapies etc.

Comparative Studies of the Efficacy of Alternative Medicine: A Research Model from Chiropractic

by Robert Anderson

This report identifies certain issues that influenced how my colleagues and I designed an ethnographically sensitive program in 1988 to investigate the efficacy of chiropractic for the treatment of chronic low back pain. Our experience in designing research relating to the efficacy of chiropractic offers a model that can be applied to other fields of alternative medicine. Unusual features of this study are as follows:

1. *A Comparison rather than a Controlled Study*
Patients were to be randomly assigned to one of three treatment groups: chiropractic, medical, or a combination of the two. All patients had these approaches explained to them and were asked to sign consent forms. The important decision here was to provide state of the art treatment to every patient/subject rather than to set up a control group that would receive a placebo/sham treatment or no treatment at all. The inability to blind this kind of a study is a cost in terms of not being able to completely eliminate subjective biases on the part of patients. Clinicians assessing treatment effects could be blinded.

2. *High External Validity*
A key decision was to aim for external rather than internal validity. That is, each treatment group was to receive whatever combination of treatments (including psychological and nutritional) that each participating doctor considered best for the individual patient. This meant that different patients would receive somewhat different treatments, in contrast to the customary practice in clinical trials of limiting treatment differences to the use or non-use of a single modality. The gain in this design is that the likelihood of patient improvement is maximized. The loss in scientific terms is that where efficacy is demonstrated, one cannot pinpoint any one aspect of the treatment regimen (such as a kind of spinal adjustment) as efficacious in itself. In that sense, internal validity is low.

3. Varied Outcome Measures

For an objective, comprehensive, sensitive, and clinically applicable evaluation of the proposed treatments, we planned to document outcome measures on a hierarchy of five different levels of efficacy. Thus, treatment effects were defined so as not to be limited to changes in the signs and symptoms of disease, as so often is the case in randomized controlled clinical trials.

A. *Anatomic-Physiologic*

Flexion-extension, lateral bending and range-of-motion measures of the lumbo-pelvic spine plus the degree of straight-leg raising were to record changes in the biomechanical efficiency of the spine. A visual analog scale would be used to measure levels of pain.

B. *Functional*

Standardized questionnaires were to be used to measure levels of daily life functioning. These were to be (i) the Oswestery Back Pain Disability Questionnaire to assess difficulty in performing daily-life functions, and (ii) the McGill Pain Questionnaire to assess perceptions of pain.

C. *Patient Satisfaction*

The extent to which each patient was pleased or not pleased with the perceived quality of care was to be elicited by means of a nine-item forced choice satisfaction scale.

D. *Financial*

Cost and utilization records were to be kept on medication use, days lost from work, days in treatment, number of treatment visits, number of treatment encounters, and total dollars billed for goods and services.

E. *Political-Economic*

The conduct of this trial was to demonstrate that an alternative form of medicine could attract the large amount of funding that would be required. It did (at U.S.$ 350,000.00). It was also to demonstrate that a mainstream medical center was willing and able to provide a setting for the anticipated program. At the final moment, prior commitments by the medical center authorities were repudiated, the funding grant had to be cancelled, and it took five years to restart the project on a smaller scale.

My Personal View on Central Aspects of Methodology of Alternative Therapies Research

by Toke Barfod

The INRAT seminars have helped me to clarify my views on many things regarding alternative therapies. For example, that whether a therapy is used or not, and whether it should be supported by government money or not, is not only a matter of proven effect or not. It is a matter of habit, values, money, side-effects, the judged probability of the rationality behind the therapy etc. However, here I will present my view on investigations of whether a therapy has effect or not.

I believe that:
- every scientific biomedical method has its own biases and limitations;
- if possible, any therapy should be investigated by a range of methods. It should be investigated by experimental, double-blinded methods as well as some less intervening methods that investigate the effectiveness of a therapy in daily practice away from experimental circumstances. This is exceedingly well done with medical therapies, and it should happen to selected alternative therapies as well;
- randomised, double-blind, placebo-controlled clinical trial is a very rigorous method and therefore one of our strongest tools in the evaluation of the efficacy of therapies;
- perhaps some doctors are too focused on randomised, double-blind, placebo-controlled trials, and some alternative therapists certainly are;

And to me, it is common sense that:
- some therapies work less, when they are performed as part of a scientific experiment. Things like the healing power of love, for example, may be hard to produce when a sceptic is watching;
- sometimes randomisation is not possible for ethical reasons. And the principle is biased in disfavour of therapies that work less if they are not deliberately chosen;
- sometimes double-blinding is not possible if the active ingredients are

easily visible. And the method is biased in disfavour of therapies that rely on the patient's and the therapist's knowledge about whether (or which) a treatment is given;
- sometimes placebo-treatments are hard to construct if a therapy is composed of many interacting active ingredients that are not precisely specified;
- sometimes the effects of a therapy are more psychological or social than physical, and therefore cannot be measured with physical instruments.

So we should be happy that we already have other scientific biomedical methods:
- randomisation between two active therapies;
- observational methods used in quality assurance, medical technology assessment, and healthservices research;
- doubleblind methods with open therapeutic guidance and single-blind methods;
- component control trials, where one of the many active ingredients are omitted from the control-treatment in order to explore its relative importance for the therapy;
- trials with a no-treatment control group;
- qualitative methods that may be able to detect therapeutic effects that are not physical.

Methodological Problems

by Christian Borchgrevink

The doubleblind randomised controlled clinical trial has been the golden standard in therapeutical research. This is probably true when it comes to evaluate new drugs, but it is obviously not suitable if you want to find out if surgery is better than medical treatment in a certain disease. If you cannot carry out a controlled trial doubleblind or singleblind, it is of utmost importance that the person who evaluates the effect in the two groups is "blinded".

We have carried out research in homeopathy using the doubleblind technique. This technique tests the effect of homeopathic drugs in certain potencies, but does not test the effect of a single remedy. Using this method, the possible beneficial effect of the 1.5 to 2-hour long first interview is excluded. If with a homeopathic treatment you mean both the interview and the homeopathic drug, testing the effect can be controlled but not double- or singleblind.

How should the control group be treated in a study on the effect of acupuncture? SHAM acupuncture? TNS? Inactive TNS? No extra treatment besides the standard? Sceptics to acupuncture would demand SHAM acupuncture. In this way the patient will (or may) be blinded. To blind the acupuncture will be extremely difficult. But is SHAM acupuncture a real placebo treatment, a totally inactive procedure? We have carried out studies in acupuncture using real acupuncture, SHAM acupuncture and untreated controls, with the effect that SHAM acupuncture lay somewhere between real acupuncture and untreated controls. But whether this effect is a placebo effect or also a certain specific effect, we cannot say.

In a controlled study on the effect of acupuncture in stroke patients, the control group received the standard rehabilitation treatment (supposed to be optimal). The acupuncture group did significantly better in several parameters, and the effect lasted at least one year (showing that the "optimal" treatment was not optimal). Whether the effect in the acupuncture group was due to the specific effect of the acupuncture or a placebo effect by the acupuncturist, we cannot say. But for the patients who improved, this is an academic question. Instead of testing the effect of acupuncture, maybe we should say: We test the effect of being treated by an acupuncturist, which includes the specific effect of the needles, the expectations of the patient for the treatment and the personality of the acupuncturist.

Psychographics. Life-Style and Complementary Medicine

by Adrian Furnham

This paper (see Furnham, this volume) will concentrate on two related methodologies concerned with the assessment of:
A) lifestyle and values
B) beliefs and attitudes

A: Lifestyles and values concerns in the market research technique of psychographics.

The paper will examine:
1. the history and background of psychographics
2. different, currently used descriptive styles (e.g. VALS)
3. advantages and disadvantages of psychographic descriptions
4. the application of psychographics to shopping for health
5. speculations on the relationship between psychographics and alternative therapies

B: Health beliefs and attitudes concerns the use of standardized psychometric questionnaires and interviews.

This paper will concentrate on specific issues related questionnaire research in alternative therapies.
1. the relationship between self-report and behaviour: do attitudes and belief questionnaires relate to health-related behaviours?
2. do "personality" variables predict use of alternative medicine?
3. can we use questionnaires developed in one country in another?
4. how honest are people in responding to questionnaires?
5. what do questionnaire studies tell us about why people choose alternative practitioners?

Various books and papers written by the author will be critically discussed. The criticisms of the post-modernist, post-empiricist movement will also be considered.

Diagnosis, Indication, Motivation

by Palle Gad

At the beginning of any treatment (therapy), sometimes at the start of any contact between client and therapist, at least three factors will constitute the situation and be of importance for the outcome: diagnosis, indication and motivation.

In my experience very few alternative therapists have realized the existence and importance of making a distinction between these three concepts. I find that in research in alternative (as well as in established) medicine the distinction, or the lack of it, may be one crucial qualification.

Diagnosis
The term 'diagnosis' covers what the problem is about, what 'Nature' brings in. It may mean a fully understood nosological entity, or a vague symptom or even a complaint; it is a word or term that the patient puts forward to the doctor/ therapist.

Indication
'Indication' is the result of professional skill and consideration: what can be done (examinations, tests, interventions or even expectation), which possibilities are available, what can be seen in favour and what counts against. In surgery and other parts of established medicine, the term contra-indication appears in any serious consideration before making the decision to act (operate) or not. Benefits, risks and costs should always be taken into consideration.

Motivation
'Motivation' is a concern of the patient alone. And the professional will never be able to know what brought his patient to him. The patient will often be under influence (inspiration) of family members, friends, etc. Here too, knowledge or expectations about benefits, risks and costs will play important roles. The therapist has to meet the ethical challenge to discern between the professional information needed by the patient and his own personal (private?) preferences; his advice will make an impact on the motivation. But in principle it is solely a matter for the patient and should be respected as such.

Questions for Research on Alternative Therapies

by Elisabeth Hsu

My questions are:

1. As many drawbacks as a quantitative assessment of treatment has (double-blind tests, etc.), it is not sensible to dismiss it altogether for the evaluation of all alternative therapies. In which instances is it sensible to apply it?

2. A frequently mentioned drawback of conventional treatment evaluation is that it is directed at investigating a method, but is healing always grounded in method? If illness management and recovery is viewed as a life process say, like aging, which science could sensibly account for it and evaluate it?

3. What do people talk about who speak of auras, prana, qi, etc.? Does treatment evaluation of alternative therapies have to take account of their conceptualisations of man and the universe and the language they use to speak about it? Why bother to understand these languages for treatment evaluation?

4. Considering that the institutionalisation, standardisation, and professionalisation of medical knowledge actually affects the modalities of knowing of alternative therapists, and that the professionalisation of alternative therapies actually leads to their adjustment to Western biomedical standards, treatment evaluation that takes account of the degree of professionalisation of alternative therapies is yet another way in which the biomedical establishment exerts its hegemony. Under which conditions can such a treatment evaluation be acceptable to alternative therapists?

An Integrative Methodology?

by Helle Johannessen

The discussion on research methodology in alternative therapy seems to be stuck in old patterns with different parties clinging to each their own favorite saying. 'Pros' as well as 'cons' seem to defend well known (and worn out) ideas and neglect the complexity of documented knowledge published in well respected research journals within the past years.

Orthodox doctors tend to demand randomized, blinded, controlled trials as the only valid documentation of therapeutic efficacy. Others argue that this research design cannot be used in alternative therapy. The argument goes that alternative therapy is based on fundamental assumptions of the human being as a multidimensional being in process, and that treatments are aimed at
1) more dimensions than traditional controlled clinical trials can handle, and
2) unique processes of development in each person, which cannot be documented by methods of generalisation and statistical processing.

Central problems seem to be
a) that there is no congenial understanding of the concepts of 'disease', 'treatment', 'healing' and 'evaluation', and
b) that there is a tendency to argue for the use of a methodology including one or the other research method.

It should be obvious, that different conceptual constructions of disease and healing call for different kinds of evaluation, and that several methods can supplement each other in a methodology including one and the other research method.

Controlled, blinded, randomized trials can be used in so far as they are compatible with the form of treatment studied. It may not be possible to do a placebo control, but patients may be their own controls, or a control group may receive the best known treatment in general use, or no treatment. It may not be possible to blind patient and practitioner, but the data processors may be blinded. The clinical trial can be modified to meet specific characteristics of a given form of treatment.

But other kinds of evaluation must be involved whenever treatments are aiming at more than a purely physio-chemical effect. The efficacy of a given treatment on the patients feeling of sorrow or social isolation cannot be measured in the physiological or chemical features of the body. It may be revealed through conversations, registration of behaviour, and to some extent by questionnaires. Even though the results of such investigations may not be presentable in diagrams or statistical processing, it is usually possible to document some general tendencies and principles in the studied population.

In addition, it may prove useful to evaluate any given treatment's effect on the economy of the patient, the practitioner and the state/insurance; it's effect on environment (in production as well as consumption), on health culture, on personal competence of the individual, etc. The potential parameters of effect are numerous. What is essential is that the method used is adequate for researching the parameters of effect in focus. Furthermore, the evaluation of any treatment should never be confined to measurements in the physioanatomical body. The effect of any treatment always involves more than physio-chemical changes in the body and is not fully understood if we pretend it is not (i.e., economy and ecology are always involved).

Much would be gained if we stopped arguing what method is The Right One. The simple answer is: None of them alone – but all of them together. Supplementing each other, qualitative and quantitative studies may provide estimation of a variety of 'values' and 'qualities' of a given form of treatment. A complex methodology may reveal 'significance' of this treatment in several respects: for the patient (physically, socially, emotionally and culturally), for the practitioner, for society, for culture and for nature.

A necessary step toward the creation of a complex methodology for therapy research is to define the explanatory potentials and limits of a variety of proposed/used methods. What can be explained and evaluated in traditional clinical trials – and by what criteria? What can be evaluated by the use of participant-observation – and by what criteria? What can be explained and evaluated by qualitative interviews, or economical estimations?

By answering such questions a multi-disciplinary research methodology for evaluation of therapy could be established. We do not have to invent anything new, but rather to organize methods already known but not yet connected in an overall methodology.

Methodological Perspectives

by Laila Launsø

There is increasing pressure on alternative treatments to document effects by using the randomized double-blind controlled clinical trial. We need more discussions and reflections on the possibilities and limitations for using this method.

One of the obvious problems in using the randomized double-blind controlled clinical trial is the reduction of a *treatment* to a single *technique*. We need more clarification on ontological and epistemological issues related to concepts such as disease, treatment, effects and "effective" treatment. Talking about "effective" treatment, do we need to take into account negative effects of treatments in relation to the environment?

I think we need a research which gives priority to a move towards the following:

Theme (objectives)	actions, processes, subjects
Relations	internal motives, intentions, norms, values, interests
Relationship	action as expression of subjective conditions
Theory	theories expressed in a context-dependent language
Methodological paradigm	the subject-oriented paradigm
Values	subject-dependent, subject-object relation is integrated, valueladen
Utilization	communicative, internal regulation
Concepts regarding illness and disease	understanding, interpretation, listening, learning, action, development
"Settings"	the natural milieu as settings

To research the *conditions for the healing process*, interdisciplinary considerations of qualitative and process-oriented natural sciences and human science approaches are both necessary and challenging in my vision.

Alternative therapy is obviously a very complex research field where input and output cannot be related easily. We are researching a field where treatments cannot be standardized but must be adapted to the individual. The situation calls for the development of "a science of the unique or the concrete", that is "context-dependent science" including the treatment model, the concrete treatment approach and effects defined in a very broad way. It is my earnest belief that understanding and action-oriented modes of research are needed in this science. These modes of research require "hands-on research" by the researcher, and demand that subjectivity and the subject's socio-cultural environmental contexts are taken into consideration.

The different modes of research produce different types of knowledge and represent different knowledge systems. The descriptive and explanatory modes of research produce objectivistic knowledge; the understanding mode of research produces hermeneutical knowledge; and the action-oriented mode of research produces praxeological knowledge. In order to understand healing processes we need to give priority to producing knowledge related to understanding and action-oriented modes of research.

Science and Communication Paradigms, Models and Communicative Strategies in the Philosophy of Medicine and Health Care Sciences

by Hjördis Nerheim

My presentation at the seminar is based on my book of 1995. This abstract is, therefore, also an abstract of the central argument of that book. My topic is the relation between the experimental and quantitative methods of bio-medical research and the qualitative methods that we may also find in bio-medical research but are more at home in the humanities.

I do not discuss the plethora of quantitative or qualitative methods, or the "sense" or senses in which the qualitative methods are methods. But I do offer a defence of qualitative research. My defence is not of qualitative research as opposed to quantitative research. That would hardly make sense. Nor is it a defence of qualitative research as a legitimate addition to quantitative research. My defence of qualitative research is that it is presupposed by quantitative research, so that for quantitative research to disregard qualitative research is to disregard its own foundations.

Qualitative research is grounded on *Verstehen* (hermeneutics). What I try to show, then, is that the procedures of quantitative research are also grounded on Verstehen. Experimental and quantitative bio-medical research loses both its guiding light and its raison d'etre if it cuts its connections to hermeneutics, that is, to the understanding of (or: to the constant striving to understand) what it is to be a human being in a human world. If that is so, then the challenge to the philosophy of the health care sciences is to be found where the quantitative methods of bio-medicine intersect with the qualitative methods of nursing, or, where bio-medical research intersects with medical care.

The language of natural science, and so of medicine as a natural science, can be regarded as having been moulded to serve "one-way communication", that is, to tell the addressee, e.g. the patient, how things are. The language of hermeneutics can be regarded as having been moulded to serve "two-way communication", that is, the working out of a mutual understanding between two speakers, e.g. the doctor and the patient, of a situation that comprises both of them. The thesis that the natural sciences, no less than the humanities, find their grounding in hermeneutics, has as its corollary the thesis that the language of *one-way communication* is grounded on the language of two-way communication.

Where medical practice is ruled by one-way communication, and understanding itself to be tied to it by its own technology, instruments and routines, it will show all the signs of an estranged practice.

In *Part I* I try to show that this estrangement can be transcended. The way out lies in a deeper understanding of the very same natural science that fostered the estrangement in the first place. The way out, that is, lies in a deeper understanding of their own practices by the practitioners of natural science.

In *Part II* I try to show that hermeneutics is to be understood, not as one method among others, but rather as a working out of the critique of the estranged science that I discuss in Part I. Through this working out, the foundations of hermeneutics are themselves revealed.

In *Part III* I present a few case studies, or exemplary tales, that serve to reveal the "unspoken premises" of biomedical research. Biomedical research is to be seen as situated within medical practice. And it can be shown that medical practitioners have a deep and implicit understanding of their own practice that, more often than not, escape their own professed understanding of it. Where they profess to be technicians, working on the basis of a technologically understood natural science, they may, on a deeper analysis, reveal themselves to be practicing within an understanding of their own practice that can only be described as hermeneutical.

References

Nerheim, Hjördis
1995   *Vitenskap og Kommunikasjon: Paradigmer, modeller, og kommunikative strategier i helsefagenes vitenskapsteori,* Scandinavian University Press: Oslo, Stockholm, Copenhagen, Oxford, Boston.

Central Aspects of Methodology in Research on Alternative Therapies

by Phillip Nicholls

1. The Healing Process Itself
Still largely the case that 'Natura sanat, non medicina'. How does the body organize healing in terms of time and space? How is this related to consciousness and perception, and in what ways (if at all) are 'the self' (and other selves) articulated to this process? Ultimately, perhaps, some ontological questions here.

2. Research on Research
What are the appropriate methodologies for evaluating alternative therapies? The randomised doubleblind controlled clinical trial is not (always or ever?) appropriate, because it de-individualizes, de-personalizes and helps to reproduce existing hierarchies of epistemological credibility in medicine. An approach which embraces (celebrates) the inter-subjectivity of therapist and patient (rather than screening it out), and is sensitive to qualitative and life-enhancing outcomes, as well as quantitative effects, might be more appropriate. Feminist-inspired autobiographical approaches (the location of researcher and researched in the research process as integral elements which affect and are affected by it) have made a welcome contribution to the development of sociological methods: they may provide a useful model for research in alternative therapy.

3. Cure and Care
In an era of largely chronic illness, it may be appropriate for research to focus more on the processes of care delivered by alternative healers than on curative outcomes. Involving the patient in the healing process and providing her with ways of managing (taking control of) illness and disease is important in so far as it is concerned with the quality rather than the quantity of lived experience.

4. *Costs*

In relation to the generalized crisis in healthcare budgets which are now characteristic of the advanced industrial democracies – some careful comparison of relative 'inputs and outputs' of conventional versus alternative treatments of particular conditions would be important political ammunition. Begs a few questions (e.g., what is appropriate research for alternative medicine? – see 2 above), but let the health economists have a systematic go anyway on obvious candidates like back pain, allergies, dermatological conditions.

5. *Politics and Action for Health*

Take the opportunity in research to connect the holistic philosophy which characterizes the therapeutic encounter in alternative therapy to a more radical politics. 'Minds' and 'Selves', as G. H. Mead observed (1934), exist in 'Society'. Emotional states which have bodily consequences are (often) socially located, and where e.g. stress, anxiety, fear and uncertainty are the product of political failures (unemployment, poverty, poor housing, the degradation and contamination of food chains and of the environment etc.), it should be pointed out. For individuals these are personal troubles; for therapists and researchers they should also be seen as social problems.

6. *Professional Regulation*

Continue to examine the organization and delivery of alternative medicine, with particular regard to the development of internal mechanisms of professional regulation and accreditation and the elaboration of codes of ethics. Healers or entrepreneurs? The two, of course, are not exclusive, but something needs to provide quality assurance for the public.

References

Mead, G. H.
   1934   *Mind, Self and Society*, Chicago University Press: Chicago.

Methodology in Complementary Medicine (CM) – A Viewpoint

by Bruno Riek

"...after 5 years, the office (of alternative medicine – OAM/NIH) has yet to show that any alternative medicine works or does not work. Some academic scientists say the office follows questionable standards and is awarding for dubious studies." These harsh words on the front page of *The N.Y. Times* (17 June, 1996) seem to address not only the OAM but research in the field of CM in general.

According to the U.S. Congress, Office of Technology Assessments (1994), it is estimated that only 10-20% of all applied procedures in medicine have been tested in view of their security and efficacy according to scientific criteria. Could it be that the standards applied to CM are different? – According to David St. George a *"review of research designs in three leading (school) medical journals found only 16% of published articles over a 10-year period were randomized trials. Of the other 84%, 49% were observational cohort studies, 14% were uncontrolled trials, and 21% were nonrandomized control trials..."* (Research into CM, Advances, 1994, 10(3): 59-60).

Many arguments have been brought forward why randomization in CM is often not possible. Two of them, I believe, are underestimated. The first refers to the relationship between the physician and the patient. Still today may be true what Paracelsus demanded centuries ago: *"Apart from the observation of nature the treatment needs to be guided by compassion and love to the patient. This is not only the ethical and moral obligation of the physician but a presupposition of successful treatment."*[1] How can it be that under these conditions a physician will treat (or accept the possibility to treat) his/her patient with placebo or in other ways than according to his/her convictions.

The second argument refers to the patient. How can we expect him/her to mobilize all the fighting power to change lifestyle, to meditate, to visualize the

---

[1] ...wo nun der arzt in solcher lieb und barmherzigkeit nicht geneigt ist, so wird er beraubt desjenigen so im zu wissen zusteht (S. Johne, 1995: Naturphilosophie – Ursprung und Bezugspunkt der Naturheilkunde, in: *Aerztezeitschrift für Naturheilverfahren*: 36(12): 916).

healing process and at the same time request the participation in a RCT where the treatment may be different that which he/she is convinced of?

To overcome these difficulties I suggest putting more weight on *outcomes studies* which measure the impact of medical interventions experienced by the patient. Such studies will move some research from the laboratory to the patient, where the focus should be. The requested cooperation is certainly more acceptable to the (future) patient than being randomized.

Prof. E. Ernst has reviewed 14 such studies (Forschende Komplementärmedizin 1995, 2: 326-9). He found among other things that *"patient's perceived effectiveness is generally encouraging: the majority of those using complementary forms of treatment experience some benefits from it. This, however, does not tell us whether such remedies are specifically effective (superior to placebo or sham intervention) or work through nonspecific placebo effects. The only way to find out is to conduct RCTs."*

In my view outcomes studies need control groups or previously accepted general standards (possibly published by health insurance companies). If there is no comparison, results of clinical studies risk being interpreted according to the researcher's and the reader's previously set viewpoint. Blinding will often not be possible and randomization must be limited to areas where it is suited best. Instead of measuring the placebo effect as a separate, almost disturbing factor, it should be optimized by the treating physician. Many other effects caused by complementary treatments are also unspecific (diet, trust, will to recover etc.). Does it matter to a satisfied patient?

Methods about the Living

by Kirsten Skjerbæk

The positivist tradition has made a virtue out of separating the scientist from the explored object. This has meant that it is possible to let the scientist stand outside of the explored activity as a passive spectator to the actions going on between the experiment and the phenomena to be explored. From the viewpoint of theory of science the positivist tradition has been 'punched out' long ago, but in the scientific world there are still bastions where it is retained. This applies especially in medical and agricultural science. It is most striking that it is in these two areas that there is one common denominator: the chemical industry! – that represents power and money.

All of us today have grown up within the influence of positivist-materialistic natural science. This has left its mark in our whole way of thinking; marks so deep that we do not normally think about the fact that we have a special way of thinking. Furthermore, it means that we carry out a lot of different actions in daily life, and in our scientific undertakings, without thinking about the underlying set of theories; the particular lifeview; the particular paradigm.

I will consider here, especially, our lifeview: how we look at life, the living. In natural science we have different disciplines dealing with the living organism: organic chemistry, biology, biochemistry etc. These are, however, viewing the living as merely ongoing processes which are just more complicated, more extensive and have larger molecules than the nonliving – the inorganic.

We evade the living as if it were just a variety of the dead. We have a theory that says that the living has arisen from inorganic matter. We do not understand the living as being totally different from inorganic matter. We do not regard life to be something uniquely on its own. If I am going to examine the *quality* and the nutritional value (i.e., the quality of life) of a carrot, I will analyse the *quantum* of its differing contents. I will find the carrot to be good nourishment if it contains a number of particular elements (vitamins, etc.) and little or no contaminants (heavy metals, pesticides, etc.). But nobody thinks about the *quality* of the essential nutritional constituents. We have, actually, no real idea about the meaning of quality. For most people vitamin-C and ascorbic acid will be the same. We cannot grasp that there should be a *qualitative* difference between vitamin-C extracted from a rosehip and the synthetically produced ascorbic acid.

We have no idea of the living because we have no clear view of the life-force itself. It is not included within our paradigm. If we seek to develop methods to investigate the living, then immediately our paradigm becomes very important, because it lies outside the 'norm'. The "picture creating" methods which are developed within biodynamic agriculture, and the anthroposophical medicine production systems, are developed to tell us something about living processes. They are developed to make it possible for us to experience something of the living activity – the life-force – within living organisms. But, of course, these methods imply and include a specific paradigm which sets up ideas and theories about this living activity within living organisms. At the same time it *includes* the scientist as playing an active role within the scientific activity and process; the scientist is the one who acknowledges everything about the processes occurring within the object matter; within him/herself and between him/her and the phenomena.

Some Personal Remarks on Methodology in Research on Alternative or Complementary Therapies

by Wolfgang Weidenhammer

In general there is no doubt about the need for research on Complementary Medicine.

But which methods are appropriate?

First step
I think the scientific community within Alternative Medicine will accept that – as a first step – there is still a need for describing very extensively
- what kind of patients
- with which set of diagnosis are treated
- with which therapies (single or a whole bundle)
- within which therapeutical setting (in- or outpatient)
- by whom (medical discipline, level of education on special methods)
- with which success (immediate and long-term results)

The instrument of quality management enriched by scientific methods offers the possibility to investigate the above aspects.

For the in-patient situation the Münchener Modell has been practicing this technique for several years and is now establishing the structure to do this for outpatients as well.

Second step
The second step should deal with the question of proving the evidence of the applied therapies by demonstrating their effectiveness or the patients' benefit.

The findings of step one should help to create clear questions or hypotheses. It is absolutely necessary to check out the appropriateness of various methodologies (like case series, long-term studies, non-randomized comparisons). The

Golden standard – the randomized clinical trial – should also be discussed concerning the external validity of results of trials of this type.

Third step
Explanation and interpretation of the findings should form the third step. Within the frame of theories which claim to do this it is very important to discuss the choice of criteria to measure the success of therapies from the Complementary/Alternative point of view. Especially for chronically ill patients it should be crucial to investigate the psychological influences (for example, different belief systems) on disease and health care. Other topics are the importance of the placebo effect, the patients' attitudes towards complementary medicine or the question of which factors determine patients' satisfaction after all.

INRAT
– a network project
for research on alternative therapies

by Helle Johannessen, Jørgen Østergård Andersen, Bent Eikard, Palle Gad, Erling Høg, Laila Launsø, Søren Gosvig Olesen

International Network for Research on Alternative Therapies (INRAT) has existed from February 1993 to December 1996 on the basis of a grant of 500,000 kroner per year received from the State Research Council for the Humanities. INRAT has during this period taken initiative to six types of activities:
1) development of theoretical work in a cross-disciplinary core group
2) annual international seminars on research on alternative therapy
3) publication of papers presented at the international seminars
4) establishment of a database for the field
5) seminars for Danish researchers and research students
6) general dissemination of information

The following will present information about each of the activities (1-6); important changes in relation to the original project description (7); themes and reflections resulting from the theoretical questions discussed during the project's activities (8); and future network activities inspired by INRAT (9).

1. Development of theoretical work in a cross-disciplinary core group

The project was led by a cross-disciplinary core group that has been engaged throughout in continuous internal theoretical discussions. These have been discussions of the themes raised at the project's international seminars as well as by the individual members' research and theoretical reflections.

Members of the core group:
Jørgen Østergård Andersen (ethnographer)
Bent Eikard (medical doctor) – vice-chairman 1995, chairman 1996

Palle Gad (medical doctor) – vice-chairman 1996
Erling Høg (anthropology student) – secretary 1994-96
Helle Johannessen (anthropologist) – scientific secretary 1993-95, coordinator 1995-96
Laila Launsø (sociologist)
Søren Gosvig Olesen (philosopher) – chairman 1995
Frants Staugaard (medical doctor)
Bobby Zachariae (psychologist)

Core group meetings
A total of nine workshops dealing with theoretical discussions were held. Each lasted 2 days.
    1993 – 2 workshops
    1994 – 2 workshops
    1995 – 3 workshops
    1996 – 2 workshops

During these workshops, members of the group presented their own articles and papers as well as those of others for consideration for the common discussions. We also visited and heard presentations at the following treatment centres in Denmark: Lotus Centre (Frørup), The Health Centre (Rudkøbing), The Ayurvedic Clinic at Rørvig Folk High School, The Growth Centre (Nørre Snede).

In addition, the core group and the project Executive Board held several day-long meetings and telephone meetings of an administrative character.

2. Annual international seminars on research on alternative therapy

Yearly seminars have been held, each lasting 2 days and concentrating on a specific theme.
    1993 Nordic research on alternative therapies (55 participants)
    1994 Body and nature in alternative therapy (60 participants)
    1995 Communication in and about alternative therapy (34 participants)
    1996 Lifestyle, medical paradigms and alternative therapy (44 participants)

Participants at three of the seminars were invited researchers and practitioners, while one seminar (1994) was open and widely announced. Participants represented a broad cross-section of disciplines, mostly researchers within the social sciences and humanities from Europe and USA but mainly from Denmark and the other Scandinavian countries.

In connection with the first seminar, we received a grant of Nkr. 25,000 from NORFA to cover travel expenses for participants from outside Denmark.

In addition to the exchange of knowledge and theoretical discussions, the seminars were also used to establish networks. Some researchers have participated in several or all of the seminars and through them established contacts that in some cases have led to concrete cooperation.

3. Publication of papers from the international seminars

INRAT has published, in cooperation with Odense University Press, a four-volume series *(Studies in Alternative Therapy 1-4)*, one volume for each of the four international seminars.

Studies in Alternative Therapy 1. Contributions from the Nordic Countries, 1994, contains 26 of the seminar's 27 papers, revised in the form of articles. The articles consist of status reports of research in each of the five Nordic countries, together with a series of examples of research within the social sciences, humanities and natural sciences concerning various forms of therapy.

Studies in Alternative Therapy 2. Body and Nature, 1995, consists of five of the seminar's six plenum presentations written in article form, together with personal reflections about the discussions in five of the seminar's seven workshops. The articles treat conceptions of body and nature in, for example, homoeopathy, natural medicine, spiritual healing, ancient China, current Western research projects and centres and schools for integrated medicine.

Studies in Alternative Therapy 3. Communication in and about Alternative Therapies, 1996, consists of 18 of the seminar's presentations in article form. The articles treat the newer theories and models for biological/biochemical communication processes in the body as explanatory models for the effects of certain alternative forms of treatment, as well as communication between patient and practitioner and communication about alternative forms of treatment between practitioners (orthodox and alternative) and researchers.

Studies in Alternative Therapy 4. Lifestyle and Medical Paradigms, 1997, was the only volume that has been sent out in a desktop version to the participants before the seminar, so that the discussions could take their point of departure in the written texts. The articles are also being published in book form. These ten articles treat the differences between the natural scientific and the hermeneutic paradigms and the lifestyle concept in relation to alternative therapies. For one of the articles, the core group invited Mary Ryan-Thorup, Ph.D., who participated in three of the seminars, to present a personal reflection on the method discussions from INRAT's seminars and publications.

With the publication of volume four in the INRAT series we will send the complete 4-volume set, at INRAT's expense, to relevant research libraries and institutions in Denmark:
Institute for Anthropology (CU), Department of Ethnography (Moesgaard), Institute for Social Pharmacy (DSH), DIKE, Committee for Health Information, Institute for Sociology (CU), Institute of Philosophy, Pedagogy and Rhetoric (CU), Centre for Research and Knowledge on Unconventional Cancer Treatment, The Nordic Health High School (Gothenberg), The Danish National Library of Science and Medicine (UB2), Centre for Humanistic Health Research (AAU), Institute for Psychology (AAU), Psychology Laboratory (CU), Danish Institute for Public Health, Institute for Social Medicine (Panum), Institute for Public Health (Panum).

4. Establishment of a database for the field

During the course of the whole project, references to relevant publications have been registered in an electronic database. The literature database contains some 1000 references, primarily related to research on alternative therapies in the fields of social science and the humanities, but also some Nordic literature on clinical research. Also researchers and projects having to do with alternative therapy have been registered in so far as those involved have so requested. The database contains brief information about 48 researchers and 30 research projects.

The database has been established through the use of the FileMaker program and is distributed without charge in electronic form upon request. It is also possible to download it without charge from INRAT's WWW home page: http://inet.uni-c.dk/~inrathj

5. Seminars for Danish researchers and research students

Two of the core group members were Danish delegates to *COST Action B4, Unconventional Medicine*, under the European Commission. In this connection, four one-day seminars were held for Danish members of this EU action. At these seminars, current and planned Danish research projects were presented and discussed. There were approximately 25 participants at each seminar.

6. General dissemination of information

In response to public demand and the large amount of information we have received about literature, symposia and other activities regarding alternative therapy, INRAT has since December 1994 published five small newsletters (December 1994, August 1995, February 1996, August 1996 and December 1996). These newsletters have been sent to almost 400 persons on the network's address list and are also publicly available on INRAT's WWW home page.

In addition, INRAT's secretariat continually answered individual requests concerning alternative therapy on the basis of the database and the information material that was received. The need for dissemination of information proved to be a far greater and more demanding task than was originally assumed.

7. Important changes in relation to the original project description

The most important changes in the project have been made in relation to the project's organization and infrastructure.

Expansion of the secretariat
Four advanced students of anthropology have been added to the secretariat as assistants (one in 1994, three in 1995), thereby increasing the administrative capacity significantly. The cost of student assistance was financed by a grant of DKK. 25,000 from Director and Mrs. Danielsen's Fund, and by converting some of the working hours originally budgeted for the project's scientific secretary to those of an ordinary secretary (12 scientific personnel hours to 24 student hours).

Constituting the core group structure
The project's core group chose its chairman and vice-chairman in December 1994, and at the same time reformulated the position of scientific secretary to that of coordinator. In November 1995, an independent editorial group was established for the remaining two publications.

Expansion of information media
To meet the need for dissemination of information, the INRAT project has grad-

ually expanded its information infrastructure from originally to include:
- cross-disciplinary core group workshops
- international seminars
- publication of papers from the seminars
- database

to also include:
- one-day seminars for those in Denmark interested in research on this area
- circulation of a newsletter in both printed and electronic media
- establishment of a WWW home page with information about INRAT; the project's newsletter; INRAT's database with instructions about how it can be read and downloaded; texts for the method discussion; and 'hyperlinks' to other WWW pages related to research in alternative therapy.

8. Themes and reflections in INRAT

Nordic research on alternative medicine
To the first seminar were invited Nordic researchers that worked with research in alternative medicine in order to establish a forum with insight into the extent of Nordic research in this area and to facilitate an exchange of experience among the researchers. The Nordic contact net established here revealed a rather varied picture of the research and research strategies in each of the Nordic countries.

In Finland, a small forum of researchers has existed for about ten years, which has studied alternative forms of treatment (especially traditional Finnish forms such as bone-setting, cup-setting, sauna, massage etc.) from a socio-cultural point of view. The focus has been on the use of and rationale behind these forms of treatment in a historic perspective.

In Sweden, an extensive national investigation of alternative medicine was made at the end of the 1980s. Also this study was essentially socio-cultural in nature and included many of the alternative forms of treatment found in Sweden at that time. Since then not much has happened in Swedish research within this area. In 1996, an extensive social scientific study was started of alternative medicine in the 20th century.

In Norway, a four-year national research program on alternative medicine was established in 1993. In contrast to the research in Finland and Sweden, the Norwegian research was focused to a great degree on clinical experiments with various treatment technologies (especially homoeopathic medicine and acupuncture) and was based on the medical research tradition.

In Denmark, research has until now been dominated by researchers from the social sciences and humanities. The Danish research (like research in other countries) has tried to reveal the use of and rationale behind alternative forms of treatment, but is distinctive in its contribution to the discussion of the methodological aspects of clinical research on alternative therapy. INRAT has followed this tendency up by trying to create a forum for discussions that, with their point of departure in theories and models from the social sciences and humanities, can illuminate the relationship between therapy, therapist and patient, as well as the processes that develop in the relational space within both the alternative and conventional segments of the health-care system.

Setting boundaries and relationships: alternative contra non-alternative therapy
A common theme in the discussions of the core group and at the international seminars has been the question of what constitutes an alternative form of treatment in contrast to one that is non-alternative, orthodox or established. The term 'alternative medicine' itself says that such medicine must be an alternative to something (the non-alternative). Thus, the relationship between the two categories of medicine becomes central for understanding the patterns of the medical pluralism. The concept of alternative medicine cannot be understood without first defining what constitutes treatment that is not considered alternative. By making a separation between a cultural, a social and a technical level, the alternative status can be differentiated.

On the cultural level, different basic concepts of the body, health processes and medical needs can be discerned. The medical establishment traditionally focuses on measurable aspects of the body, treatment and biochemical effects. Others focus on nonmeasurable aspects of the human being, such as personality characteristics, emotions and subjectively experienced phenomena that are called 'energy', 'aura', 'chakra' etc.

On the social level, there is the difference between on the one hand practitioners that enjoy official recognition and support, for example, in the form of authorization procedures and public funding of education and practice, and on the other hand practitioners and treatment that do not enjoy these privileges and in some countries are even illegal.

On the technical level, there is the difference between forms of treatment which are considered to be technical interventions that can be subjected to technological evaluation through the special research method called randomized, controlled trial (RCT), and forms of treatment which are considered to a greater degree to be complex relationships and processes that are thus difficult to reveal through a technological evaluation such as RCT.

A form of treatment termed alternative is not necessarily characterized by focus on subjective aspects of the body and the treatment, lack of official recognition and incompatibility with RCT, but often at least one of these characteristics will apply. INRAT's discussions have mostly treated questions on the cultural level. In the core group, Freudian psychoanalysis has repeatedly been a prototypical example of a form of treatment that takes its point of departure in a fundamentally different rationale than that of the medical establishment, but nevertheless had to subordinate itself or approach the dominating medical discourse in order to achieve acceptance and general recognition.

Body and nature
Basic assumptions about the body and about nature are considered to be the foundation for every therapeutic effort and have therefore been central aspects of INRAT's discussions during the first year.

A common basic assumption within alternative forms of therapy is that the body is an energy structure, and consequently energy and energy manipulation are used as explanatory factors in connection with treatment. Without having reached any kind of agreement as to these concepts' explanatory value, it became clear that one of the most essential problems connected with using the energy concept is that within alternative therapy it has another meaning than that which is common within natural science. These semantic differences contribute to communication problems between alternative therapists and those within the traditional natural and medical sciences, and the usefulness of the concept therefore becomes questionable. It could be useful to introduce other concepts (such as structure, pattern, dynamics) to explain the phenomena that are now widely referred to as energy.

Several presentations at the international seminars discussed the construction of the body within homoeopathy, showing that in this form of treatment the body is not explained as a physical-anatomical construction but as a structure consisting of energy levels, personality patterns, dispositions, tendencies and social characteristics. Although the homoeopathic picture of the body thus differs from that of traditional medicine, it is deeply anchored in Western cultural assumptions about human beings, since the different personality types are connected to specific types of work, social status etc. in well-known stereotypes of Western culture.

In order to embrace the many different constructions attributed to the body by the various therapies, we have tried to argue for a comprehension of the body as a complex field where the biological, physiological, social, mental and cultural aspects all interact at the same time and can be understood separately through analytical and therapeutic explanatory models.

Based on several of the presentations at the workshops and seminars, it also seems possible that the structuring, or creation of order, that happens during a process of treatment can be seen as a meaningful part of the treatment or therapy itself. It is obvious that much of the patient's suffering can be attributed to cultural and mental structuring, but at the same time the possibility exists that the concept of structuring can also be meaningful within a biological and physiological concept of disease.

Communication
The subject of communication is closely connected to the question of paradigms and methods in alternative therapies. A form of treatment is based on systematic knowledge that makes communication possible within its own frame of reference. Every treatment's language can thus be assumed to have a specific cultural structure common to those who use it.

Researchers within the area of health care and the treatment of illness and disease each have their own language and background of knowledge – each have their paradigm and research method as well. When they attempt to communicate, the problem is that they often do not speak the same language. To understand, use and communicate different systems of knowledge can thus be assumed to demand openness and tolerance as well as critical judgement about the validity of the insight gained.

INRAT has attempted to illuminate this problem by bringing international researchers working in the area of 'communication and alternative therapies' together for discussion, followed by publication of the research material presented. Both cross-cultural and cross-disciplinary problems were discussed, since researchers with different cultural, national as well as professional backgrounds, within both the natural and social sciences, tried to convey their research, insights and views about alternative frames of understanding.

The overall goal has been to create a network of researchers on alternative therapies, which would naturally mean improved communication among them. The means has been to create a continuing dialogue understood as the exchange of ideas, experiences and research results among the involved researchers.

INRAT has presented a wealth of communication research within alternative therapies. The communication problems investigated can be summarized as follows:
- among researchers – within and across different research traditions;
- among practitioners – within and across different treatment traditions;
- in the body – communication processes within the individual living human organism;

- with experiments to evaluate therapeutic effect through different methodological approaches;
- when social scientific cultural studies challenge natural scientific natural studies;
- with use of electronic media for the exchange of research ideas and results;
- with experiments in integration of diverse therapies in both research and practice;
- when political questions arise in a research situation.

Discussion of these questions within the research network, INRAT, has made clear the difficult conditions that exist for communication within and between alternative therapies, and also established therapy. Since communication problems are thus manifold, it would be logical to propose that the idea of communicating itself might be a central subject for future research in this area.

Paradigms and methods
Different paradigms unfold within the alternative and established medicine. This has also manifested itself in INRAT's work from the beginning. Our effort has been to examine these paradigms and their differences. We have tried to characterize the dominating paradigms within alternative medicine which views them as having a vitalistic, praxeological or holographical form, while established medicine prefers to see itself in light of a scientific ideal of a mathematical-reductionistic form, in spite of the fact that it must be said to build to a high degree on medicine and empiricism. These differences also apply on the ontological level in that the two forms of knowledge relate to different constructions of reality. In this regard we must point out that their understanding of the relationship between cause and effect and its significance are completely different. The established ideal in its extreme form seeks explanations of a mono-causal character. The opposite extreme focuses less on causality than on launching healing processes through the treated subject's own healing potential. Thus, alternative medicine differs in principle from the established ideology about fighting against and conquering illness. In reality, however, both the established and the alternative sectors can comprise both forms of knowledge.

Therapy forms often combine concepts from East and West, for example, Ayurveda, as it is being introduced in the West at present. This form of therapy seeks to combine newer medical concepts and models for bodily processes (e.g. neurophysiological models for information transfer in the body) with concepts and models taken from traditional Indian texts about people and disease (e.g. concepts of doshas and karma) and newer Western models and concepts from alternative therapies (e.g. energy). Such a combination of very different concepts and models is based on an idea that they can supplement each other in a holistic understanding of the human being, illness, disease and treatment. The combination implies however significant conceptual and logical problems, since the conceptual construction refers to completely different universes of meaning.

A decisive problem for research on alternative medicine is to develop methods to reveal the differently constructed reality that is the object of alternative medicine. Most methods available to research are developed within the framework of the established ideal and are thus tailored to the corresponding ontological assumptions and to that ideal's special construction of illness, disease, treatment and effect.

Lifestyle

The concept of lifestyle became part of the INRAT discussion already in 1994. This topic was new within the research on alternative therapies. The lifestyle ideas revealed multiple meanings depending on the scientific approach and the researcher's own scientific background.

As a general point of departure you could tentatively define *lifestyle* as a way of life reflecting attitudes, beliefs and values of an individual or a group. However, it became evident that the ideas of a personal or collective lifestyle hold many potential definitions. Thus, we might see definitions along a continuum: *lifestyle* in practice as a question of personal choice versus intellectual or theoretical considerations of how a person *should* choose her or his style in life.

Possible definitions of the idea of lifestyle are, however, not limited to more tangible ideas of a personal choice in practice versus theoretical obligations regarding *the* reasonable life. The idea of 'lifestyle' holds multiple meanings as part of everyday life. The concept is defined and applied in various areas of society: especially within biomedicine, marketing, market analyses, but also in sociology, philosophy and anthropology. A specific definition depends on its purpose and aim, and how one perceives life in general. How life is perceived may also depend on the personal world view or *cultural view* of life.

The discussions within the INRAT research network showed that:
- *Lifestyle* is important for the personal way of self-definition and that this lifestyle is lived in practice in relation to a specific aesthetics and performance;
- We need empirical evidence concerning the theoretical discussions of how lifestyles influence the rise of alternative therapies and how these lifestyle factors can be distinguished concerning different therapies;
- Lifestyle within everyday postmodernism expresses a distrust toward the institutions in modern society;

- The interest in alternative therapies is a product of a certain lifestyle, seen in the light of the increasing concern for ecology, spirituality and new age philosophies;
- The personal free choice of lifestyle is an expression of an increasing individual responsibility for good health, simultaneously showing an attempt to avoid the total medicalization of human suffering;
- 'Health' is a heterogeneous concept grounded in how life is *lived*, more than how it is perceived within a rational unambiguous medical theory.

The resulting discussion of the lifestyle concept within the INRAT network involved making visible its manifold possible theoretical definitions and practical applications within humanistic and social scientific research on alternative therapies. The discussions have shown a need for further investigation of the lifestyle concept within these research traditions.

9. Network for research on alternative therapies – future perspectives

With the activities outlined above, the INRAT project has been carried out as planned. Workshops, seminars, database and publications have been realized, and theoretical discussions on the chosen themes have been carried out. Thus INRAT, as an independent project, is considered completed, and the core group is dissolved as its working committee.

In addition to carrying out the planned activities, however, the project also had the goal of *establishing a network* among researchers doing work on alternative therapies, since at the time the project started no international research milieu existed in this area. We conclude this report with an evaluation of INRAT's function in relation to this goal.

Framework for establishing personal contacts
The international seminars have without doubt been significant for establishing personal as well as professional contacts between researchers from European countries (and in a few cases also from USA).

The first seminar was characterized by participants' lack of knowledge about each other, as well as uncertainty and fear about negative reactions to their work. Several participants stated that they felt isolated and marginalized in their daily work because of their research in alternative therapies. Until now, formal frameworks for cooperation between researchers in this area have not existed, and in the their institutions many felt a common lack of respect and recognition because of the research area's marginalized status.

Many have participated in several of INRAT's seminars (some in all of them), and it has been clear that knowledge about each other's work, informal contacts, professional exchanges, cooperation and even friendships have grown from seminar to seminar. The final seminar was characterized to a great extent by feelings of friendship, collectivity and professional interconnectedness among those present – a quality that was also mentioned by the participants.

The fact that qualified persons have established connections with one another is reflected by the presence at INRAT's final seminar of representatives from the most prominent organizations and institutions within European research on alternative medicine, including: the national Norwegian program for research on alternative medicine (Oslo); Cost Action B4 on Unconventional Medicine (Brussels) – represented by the chairmanship as well as delegates from Sweden, Finland, England, Switzerland and Denmark; Research Council for Complementary Medicine (London); Münchener Model (München); Wissen Archive, Akademie für Ganzheitsmedizin (Vienna); FDZ Research Council (Denmark). In addition, most of the participants must be considered to be representatives for the European elite within social scientific and humanistic research in alternative therapies based at several European universities and other research institutions (e.g. Copenhagen University, Odense University, Aarhus University, University in Oslo, Linköping University, Ludwig-Maximillian's University, Research and Knowledge Centre for Unconventional Cancer Treatment, Royal Danish School of Pharmacy, Tromsø University, The Danish Agricultural University, Kuopio University, Witten/Herdecke University, John Moore's University, Staffordshire University, Oxford University, University of Derby, Münster University).

It can thus be said that INRAT has contributed significantly to establishment of a network for research on alternative therapies among researchers within the social sciences and humanities working in this area in Europe. INRAT delivered the framework for establishing the personal contacts necessary for professional cooperation, and this framework was filled out by qualified persons from many countries. In all justice it should be noted that in addition to INRAT and during the same period, several other European initiatives have contributed to establishing networks among researchers in this area; however, INRAT has been unique in its focus on research within the social sciences and humanities, while other initiatives have been dominated by medical research in the area.

Continuation of activities started by INRAT
As a conclusion of the final seminar, a session was held to discuss possibilities for continuing some of the activities INRAT organized during its lifetime.

Seminars

It was agreed to hold four more international seminars concerning the socio-cultural aspects of alternative medicine:

    1997 The history of alternative medicine (in Sweden)
    1998 Social and political aspects of integrated medicine (in England)
    1999 Alternative medicine and gender issues (in Denmark)
    20?? Documentation in alternative medicine (in Austria)

The future organizers requested those who had arranged INRAT's activities to provide assistance in the form of address lists, advice and guidance in regard to the practical aspects of the arrangements.

Publications

An international group was established with six members for the purpose of publishing an anthology of research on alternative medicine. This will be an independent publication (not the 5th in INRAT's series). The book is intended to be directed toward a broader audience and will therefore be produced according to more commercial principles with better marketing than INRAT's publications. These were mostly directed toward those connected with the project in one way or another.

Database

Two institutions expressed interest in continuing INRAT's database (one in Germany and one in Denmark), and an Austrian institution offered to support it on a temporary basis if necessary. Subsequently the INRAT core group has, however, decided that the INRAT database shall continue as an independent one. Rather, it is free for all interested parties to include the data in other existing databases.

Electronic network

An international working group was established to write a project description and application for funds in order to establish a formal European network of WWW home pages with information about research on alternative medicine.

The name INRAT

The participants expressed the wish to maintain the name INRAT in connection with some of the above-mentioned future activities. One argument for continuing use of the name was that it has gradually become broadly known in Europe as a mark of alternative therapy research of high quality, and that a common name is a necessary symbol of common identity for those who would join the network.

INRAT's core group has since discussed this question and reached the following conclusion: Continued use of the name INRAT requires an organizational model with a central administration which can serve as a home base for the name and the network. Since at present no possibility of such a central administration for the network exists, it is not considered feasible to continue use of the name INRAT. In the long run, it could lead to persons or events not really having anything to do with INRAT being associated with it because of the name. If a central administration were to be established, then the name could be used.

In connection with the above-mentioned future activities, INRAT's core group proposes that questions about continuity and common identity be solved in the following way:

Seminars
We propose that the first seminar should be entitled: "5th International Seminar on Research on Alternative Therapies", the next: "6th International Seminar on Research on Alternative Therapies" etc. The seminars and eventual resulting publications would then be called "ISRAT".

Publications
Since the planned future publication is to be independent, it is not considered necessary for it to carry forward a common name and identity.

Database
Since the database will not be continued as an independent database, there will be no need for continuing the name INRAT.

Electronic network
Since the planned future electronic network is a completely new project, INRAT's name is considered irrelevant in this connection.

List of Contributors

David Aldridge, Professor
Mediziniche Fakultät,
Universität Witten/Herdecke
Alfred Herrhausen Str. 50
58448 Witten, Germany
e-mail: davida@uni-wh.de

Jørgen Østergård Andersen,
Senior researcher,
Center for Kulturforskning,
Aarhus Universitet
Finlandsgade 26,
8000 Århus C, Denmark
e-mail: KULTANDERSEN@cfk.hum.aau.dk

Robert Anderson, Professor
Department of Anthropology, Mills College
5000 Mac Arthur Blvd., Oakland, CA.
94613, USA
e-mail: boba@ella.mills.edu

Barfod, Toke, MD
Grønnegade 39, st., 7100 Vejle, Denmark

Christian F. Borchgrevink, Prof., dr.med.
Institute of Family Medicine, University of
Oslo, Frederik Stangs Gate 11-13, 0264
Oslo, Norway

Søren Brier, Associate Professor
The Royal School of Librarianship,
Aalborg Branch
Langagervej 4,
9220 Aalborg Ø, Denmark
e-mail: sbr@db.dk

Bent Eikard, MD
Klostervej 8, Vemmetofte,
4640 Fakse, Denmark
e-mail: beikard@pip.dknet.dk

Adrian Furnham, Professor
Dept. of Psychology,
University College London
26 Bedford Way,
London WC1E 6BT, United Kingdom
e-mail: ucjtsaf@ucl.ac.uk

Palle Gad, M.D. surgeon, psychotherapist
Badstuen 19, Troense,
5700 Svendborg, Denmark

Erling Høg, Stud. Scient. Ant., BA
Institute of Anthropology, University of
Copenhagen, Frederiksholms Kanal 4,
DK-1220 Copenhagen K, Denmark
e-mail: erling.hoeg@anthro.ku.dk

Elisabeth Hsu, Dr.
Faculty of Oriental Studies, Cambridge
University, Sidgwick Avenue, Cambridge
CB3 9DA, U.K.
e-mail: elh25@hermes.cam.ac.uk

Helle Johannessen, mag.scient., Ph.D.
Almagervej 2, 4291 Ruds Vedby, Denmark
e-mail: inrathj@inet.uni-c.dk

Laila Launsø, Dr. scient. soc.,
Associate Professor,
Department of Social Pharmacy,
Royal Danish School of Pharmacy
Universitetsparken 2,
2100 København Ø, Denmark
e-mail: LL@charon.dfh.dk

Hjördis Nerheim, Professor
Department of Philosophy,
Tromsø University, Søndre Tollbugt 7,
9008 Tromsø, Norway

Phillip A. Nicholls, Dr.
Staffordshire University, College Road,
Stoke-on-Trent, Staffordshire ST4 2DE, U.K.

Søren Gosvig Olesen, Res. Libr., mag.art.
The Royal Library, Slotsholmen,
1016 Copenhagen K, Denmark

Dirk Richter, Dr. phil.
Westfälische Klinik für Psychiatrie
PO Box 8620, D-48046 Münster, Germany,
e-mail: d.richter @t-online.de

Bruno Riek, Dr.
Oberdorfstraße 21,
3066 Stettlen, Switzerland
e-mail: somep@dial.eunet.ch

Mary Ryan-Thorup, Ph.D., Anthropology
Leerbjerg Lod 8,
3400 Hillerød, Denmark
e-mail: mthorup@diku.dk

Kirsten Skjerbæk, Cand. Pharm.
Department of Agricultural Sciences, The
Royal Veterinary and Agricultural University,
Agrovej 10, DK-2630 Taastrup, Denmark

Ane Bodil Søgård, Lic. scient.,
Research Professor
Department of Agricultural Sciences, The
Royal Veterinary and Agricultural University,
Agrovej 10, DK-2630 Taastrup, Denmark

Nelly Tsouyopoulos, Prof. Dr.
Institut für Theorie
und Geschichte der Medizin,
Westfälische Wilhelms-Universität Münster
Waldeyer Straße 27,
48149 Münster, Germany

Wolfgang Weidenhammer, Dr. rer. biol. hum.
Projektbüro Münchener Modell des LMU
München, Ludwig-Maximilian-Universität,
Kaiserstraße 9, 80801 München, Germany